PALPATORY LITERACY

PALPATORY LITERACY

The complete instruction manual
for the 'hands on' therapist

Leon Chaitow N.D., D.O.

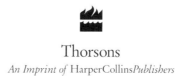

Thorsons
An Imprint of HarperCollins*Publishers*

Dedication

I wish to dedicate this book to my uncle, Boris Chaitow D.C., D.O., with profound thanks to him for teaching me so much, and to the memory of his cousin Stanley Lief D.C., D.O., the developer of Neuromuscular Technique.

Thorsons
An Imprint of HarperCollins*Publishers*
77–85 Fulham Palace Road,
Hammersmith, London W6 8JB

Published by Thorsons 1991

3   5   7   9   10   8   6   4   2

© Leon Chaitow 1991

Leon Chaitow asserts the moral right to
be identified as the author of this work

A catalogue record for this book
is available from the British Library

ISBN 0-7225-2198-7

Printed in Great Britain by The Bath Press, Bath, Avon

Contents

Structure and Function: Are they Inseparable?

One of the oldest maxims in osteopathic medicine highlights the total interdependence of structure and function; structure determines function and vice versa. Anything which causes a change to occur in structure will cause function to modify, and any functional change will result in structural change (fibrosis of muscle, alteration in length of any soft tissue, change in joint surface smoothness, are examples).

There is no way that a shortened or fibrosed muscle can function normally; there will always be a degree of adaptation, a modification from normal patterns of use, some degree of mal-coordination or imbalance in use. Similarly *all* changes in the use of a part of the body, or the whole body which vary from correct use (i.e., the way it functions) will produce alterations in structure. If posture is poor, or habitual use is incorrect (sitting cross-legged, and writing with the head tilted to one side, are common examples) structural changes will develop in response to – or in order to support and cement – these functional changes.

We can summarize factors which produce functional – and subsequently structural – change as involving overuse, misuse or abuse, which in turn can be reduced to one word: stress. Conversely, if we palpate structure and find alterations from the expected norm, we should be able to confirm related functional changes. For example if we palpate shortened or fibrosed soft tissues it should be possible to register that the area does not function optimally (for example, a shortened hamstring is palpable and the leg will not easily be lifted in a straight-leg raising test).

When we observe functional change we should readily be able to identify structural alterations which relate to this. Thus when posture or breathing function (see Chapter 8) is not as it should be, we can easily target the tissues which are most likely to carry evidence of associated structural change. On a more local scale, when skin elasticity (a function dependent on normal structure) is reduced, we know that underlying reflex change (function) is involved (see Chapter 3). Palpation and observation are as inseparable as structure and function, and this should be kept in mind during our exploration of palpatory methods.

Chapter 1

The Aims of Palpatory Literacy

It is axiomatic that practitioners who use their hands to manipulate soft or bony structures should be able, accurately and relatively swiftly, to feel, assess and judge the state of a wide range of physiological and pathological conditions and parameters, relating not only to the tissues with which they are in touch but others associated with these, perhaps lying at greater depth. The information a practitioner needs to gather will vary according to the therapeutic approach; it might be the range of motion and the feel of joint play, the relative weakness or tightness in muscles, the amount of induration, oedema or fibrosis in soft tissues, identification of regions in which reflex activity is operating, or even differences in the quality of perceived 'energy' variations in regions of the body.

Karel Lewit M.D., in his book *Manipulation in Rehabilitation of the Motor System* (Butterworths, 1987) sums up a major problem in learning to palpate when he says: 'Palpation is the basis of our diagnostic techniques [and yet] it is extremely difficult to describe exactly, in words, the information palpation provides.' With the help of numerous experts from a variety of disciplines, we will try, nonetheless, to do this, all the while keeping in mind the words of Viola Frymann D.O., (in the *1963 Yearbook of the Academy of Applied Osteopathy*): 'Palpation cannot be learned by reading or listening; it can only be learned by palpation.'

Much of this book comprises descriptions of various forms of palpation, highlighting different ways in which this may be best achieved along with numerous examples of exercises which can help in the development of perceptive exploratory skills. Of course, what we make of information derived from palpation will depend upon how it fits into a larger diagnostic picture, which needs to be built up from case-history taking and other forms of assessment. Such interpretation is naturally essential in order for treatment to have any direction; palpation is anything but an end in itself. However, interpretation of the information derived from palpation is not a major purpose of this text; the main purpose is learning to palpate. (This is not because such interpretation of information is regarded as being of only secondary importance – for it is not – but to have ventured too far into that realm would have expanded the text to an unmanageable size.)

For example, in Chapter 3, which deals with assessment of skin tone elasticity, we will discover how to make an accurate assessment of local or general areas in which there is a relative loss of the ability of the skin to stretch due to reflex activity. This section therefore deals with the art of palpation of these particular tissues in terms of this particular characteristic (elasticity, adherence). What the finding of local skin 'tightness' may mean in terms of pathological or physiological responses, and what to do about it, will also be touched on in terms of the opinion of various experts, but it is not possible to give a comprehensive survey of all possible opinions on the topic.

In other words the individual therapist will have to fit the acquired information into their own belief system and use it in accordance with their own therapeutic methodology. The aim of the book will be to help in identifying what is under our hands.

We can equate palpation with learning to make sense of some other form of information, say that relating to music. It is possible to learn to read music, to understand its structure, theory of harmony, tones and chords, and even something of the variations of the application of such knowledge to different forms of composition. However, this would not allow you to play an instrument. The instrument we play is the human body, and the development of palpatory literacy allows you to 'read' that body.

One of osteopathy's major figures, Frederick Mitchell Jr D.O. makes a different comparison when he equates the learning of palpatory literacy with that of visual literacy:

> Visual literacy is developed in visual experiences and the exercise of visual perceptions in making judgements. Visual judgements and perceptions may be qualitative or quantitative or both. Although the objectives in training the diagnostic senses do not include esthetic considerations, esthetic experiences probably are developmental in terms of visual literacy. In making esthetic value judgements one must be able to discriminate between straight lines and crooked lines, perfect circles and distorted circles.... To evaluate the level of sensory literacy, one may (also) test for specific sensory skills in a testing situation.
>
> *(Yearbook of the American Academy of Osteopathy, 1976)*

In later chapters I will suggest ways in which this can be done.

Assumptions and Paradoxes

The text of the book makes an assumption that the reader has at least a basic knowledge of anatomy and physiology, and ideally of pathology. It is necessary to emphasize that we must distinguish between what we are palpating, what we actually sense, and the way we interpret the information thus gained. It is all too easy for the practitioner (even those with wide experience) to feel what he or she 'wants' to feel, or what he or she expects to feel. A relative degree of detachment from the process of assessment is therefore helpful if not essential.

An open mind is also vital to the task of learning palpatory literacy, those practitioners with the greatest degree of 'rigidity' in terms of their training, and of the system of therapy they follow, often have the hardest time in allowing themselves to feel new feelings, sense new sensations. Those with the most open, eclectic, approaches (massage therapists are a prime example) usually find it easiest to 'trust' their senses and feelings.

The other side of this is the fact that many (by no means all) such 'open' therapists also have the poorest knowledge of anatomy/physiology and pathology against which to relate their palpatory evaluations. This paradox can only be resolved by highly-trained professionals becoming more intuitive and open, trusting that they really are sensing very subtle sensations as they open themselves to developing the delicate skills necessary for many palpatory methods; and at the same time many 'less well-trained' professionals may need to accept that there is indeed a need to add layers of knowledge, to their intuitive and nurturing talents.

Unless a practitioner is able to 'read' with the hands the information which abounds in all soft tissues, and is also able to relate this to the problems of the patient – as well as to a good deal of other diagnostic information – a great deal of potentially vital data will be missed. No one in the osteopathic field has done more to stress the importance of sound palpatory skills that Viola Frymann D.O., and we will be learning from a number of her observations as we progress through the text. She summed up the focusing of these skills, and the importance of making sense of them, when she said:

> The first step in the process of palpation is detection, the second step is amplification, and the third step must therefore be interpretation. The interpretation of the observations made by palpation is the key which makes the study of the structure and function of tissues meaningful. Nevertheless it is like the first visit to a foreign country. Numerous strange and unfamiliar sights are to be seen, but without some knowledge of the language with which to ask questions, or a guide to interpret those observations in the life and history of the country, they have little meaning to us. The third step in our study then is to be able to translate palpatory observations into meaningful anatomic, physiologic or pathologic states.
>
> (*Yearbook of American Academy of Osteopathy, 1963*)

What Other Experts Say about Palpation

Philip Greenman D.O., in his superb analysis *Principles of Manual Medicine*, summarizes the five objectives of palpation:

1. to be able to detect abnormal tissue texture;
2. to be able to evaluate symmetry in the position of structures, both tactically and visually;
3. to be able to detect and assess variations in range and quality of movement during the range, as well as the quality of the end of the range of any movement;
4. to be able to sense the position in space of yourself and the person being palpated;
5. to be able to detect and evaluate change in the palpated findings,

whether these are improving or worsening as time passes.

As will become clear, others have added more subtle but still palpable factors, such as energy variations, 'tissue memory' and emotional residues, to these basic requirements. These, though, are our major objectives in obtaining palpatory literacy.

Dr Karel Lewit, the brilliant Czechoslovakian physician who has eclectically combined so much of osteopathic, chiropractic, physical therapy and orthopaedic knowledge, states his objective in palpating the patient thus:

> Palpation of tissue structures seeks to determine the texture, resilience, warmth, humidity and the possibility of moving, stretching or compressing these structures. Concentrating on the tissues palpated, and pushing aside one layer after another, we distinguish skin, subcutaneous tissue, muscle and bone, we recognize the transition to the tendon, and finally the insertion. Palpating bone, we recognize tuborosities (and possible changes) and locate joints. Reflex changes due to pain affect all these tissues, and can be assessed by palpation; one of the most significant factors is increased tension.

We will examine Lewit's methods of ascertaining the presence of tense, tight tissues in some detail in later chapters. Gerald Cooper D.O. says:

> 'To begin to learn palpatory skill one must learn to practise to palpate bone or muscle or viscera. Gradually one learns to distinguish between a healthy muscle, a spastic muscle, and a flaccid one, and gradually one learns there is a difference in feel between a hard malignant tumor and a firm benign tumor, *Palpation cannot be learned by reading or listening, it can only be learned by palpation.*
>
> *(Academy of Applied Osteopathy Yearbook 1977,* My emphasis.)

This message is basic and vital, and many experts repeat it. Read, understand, and then practice, practice, and practice some more. It is the only way to become literate in palpation. George Webster D.O., writing in the *1947 Yearbook of the American Academy of Osteopathy* said:

> We should feel with our brain as well as with our fingers, that is to say, into our touch should go our concentrated attention and all the correlated knowledge that we can bring to bear upon the case before us....The principle employed by Dr Still [founder of osteopathy] in so carefully educating his tactile sense as he did with his Indian skeletons and living subjects, together with the knowledge to properly interpret the findings, accounted for his success over such a wide field. He had a way of letting his fingers sink slowly into the tissues, feeling his way from the superficial to the deep structures, that gave him a comprehensive picture of local as well as general pathology.

On the learning of palpatory skills, Frederick Mitchell Jr states:

> Although visual sensing of objects is done through an intervening medium (the atmosphere or other transparent material), students are rather uncomfortable with the notion that palpation is also performed through an

intervening medium (Becker said to palpate *through* your fingers, not with them). The necessity for projecting one's tactile senses to varying distances through an intervening medium must seem mystical and esoteric to many beginning students. Yet even when one is palpating surface textures the information reaches one's nervous system through one's own intervening integument. Students are often troubled by the challenge of palpating an internal organ through overlying skin, subcutaneous fascia and fat, muscle, deep fascia, subserous fascia and peritoneum.

Suspending Judgement

It is just the 'troubled' feeling towards such challenges which the exercises and advice in the text will hopefully overcome, for along with the assertion of so many experts that palpation can only be learned by palpating, there is another common theme; there must be a trusting of what is being felt, a suspension of critical judgement while the process is being carried out. Later on critical judgement may be used in interpreting what was felt, but, the process of 'feeling' needs to be done with that faculty silenced. No one has better expressed this need than John Upledger D.O., the developer of craniosacral therapy. In *Craniosacral Therapy* he states:

> Most of you have spent years studying the sciences and have learned to rely heavily upon your rational, reasoning mind. You probably have been convinced that the information which your hands can give you is unreliable. You may consider facts to be reliable only when they are printed on a computer sheet, projected on a screen or read from the indicator of an electrical device. In order to use your hands and to begin to develop them as reliable instruments for diagnosis and treatment, you must learn to trust them and the information they can give you.
>
> Learning to trust your hands is not an easy task. You must learn to shut off your conscious, critical mind while you palpate for subtle changes in the body you are examining. You must adopt an empirical attitude so that you may temporarily accept *without question* those perceptions which come into your brain from your hands. Although this attitude is unpalatable to most scientists it is recommended that you give it a trial. After you have developed your palpatory skill, you can criticize what you have felt with your hands. If you criticize before you learn to palpate, you will never learn to palpate, you will never learn to use your hands effectively as the highly sensitive diagnostic and therapeutic instruments which, in fact, they are.

Accept what you sense as real is Upledger's plea. It is an ideal motto for this exploration of palpatory skills.

Dr W.G. Sutherland, the primary osteopathic researcher into cranial motion, gave his uncompromising instruction as follows:

> It is necessary to develop fingers with brain cells in their tips, fingers capable of feeling, thinking, seeing. Therefore first instruct the fingers how to feel, how to think, how to see, and then let them touch.

(The Cranial Bowl)

**A Wide Range of
Palpatory Objectives**

As though the fears outlined by Mitchell were insufficient, or Upledger's and Sutherland's directions not difficult enough, there are also those therapists who make an assessment a short distance from the skin, although it should be clear that what they are 'palpating' is rather different from the tissues Mitchell's students were palpating.

This approach is far less indefensible than might be assumed, following the publication of the results of double blind studies into the use of Therapeutic Touch methods, in which no contact with the (physical) body is made at all. This will be discussed further in Chapter 9 where an array of methods aimed at increasing sensitivity to subtle energy patterns in detailed. Other forms of assessment involve very light skin contact, either with the palpating hand(s)/digit(s) stationary or moving in a variety of ways, and these methods will also be explored at length. Palpation of this sort often employs, as Lewit mentioned, awareness of variations in skin tone, temperature, feel and elasticity (which may reflect or be associated with altered electrical resistance) or other changes.

Some methods, such as the German system of *bindegewebsmassage* (connective tissue massage) employ a sequential examination of the relative adherence of different layers of tissue to each other, either at an interface (say between muscle and connective tissue) or above it (skin over muscle, muscle over bone and so on). Lewit too has shown the relevance of identifying changes in skin adherence over reflex areas which are active (trigger points, for example).

Recent developments – as well as the reintroduction of older concepts – have led to methods of assessment of visceral structures, both in terms of position and 'motion', and some of the methods involved will be presented. Craniosacral and zero balancing methods (among others) use the sensing of inherent rhythms, felt on the surface, to make assessments of relative physiological or pathological states, or even of 'tissue memory' relating to trauma, either physical or emotional. Variations on these methods will be examined and described together with the description of exercises which assist in developing appropriate degrees of sensitivity for their effective use.

Deeper palpation of the soft tissues, involving stretching, probing, compressing and the use of various movements and positions are all commonly employed to seek out information relating to local and reflex activity; these approaches will also be examined and explained. Such methods are frequently combined with the use of sequential assessment of the relative degree of tension (shortness) or strength of such muscles. Examination of some of the ways in which joint status can be judged from its 'end-feel', when range of motion and motion palpation are used for this purpose, add a further dimension to the art of palpation.

As mentioned above, wherever possible guidelines to enhance sensitivity will be given as the various approaches are covered. What the findings may mean will be surveyed, both in relation to obvious biomechanical changes as well as possible reflex and psychological implications. This latter element is something we should always be aware of, as there are few chronic states of dysfunction which are not overlaid (or often caused) by psychosomatic interactions. Indeed research by German connective tissue massage therapists has clearly demonstrated specific, palpable, soft tissue changes relating to particular emotional or psychological states.

The therapeutic methods involved in the practice of osteopathy, chiropractic, physiotherapy, massage therapy and a host of systems and methods associated with bodywork, have all developed individualized diagnostic methods, some of which have become universally applied and valued by other systems; in order not to upset professional sensitivities credit will be given to the system which developed particular palpatory methods wherever this is known.

Ida Rolf, the developer of structural integration through the system known as Rolfing, gave an idea of just how exciting an experience palpation can be; in her book *Rolfing: The Integration of Human Structures* she suggests that the beginner in the art of palpation should feel their own thigh (as an example). Initially, she says, this will feel 'undifferentiated', either overly dense of soft, lacking in tone, or as though large lumps were held together under the skin. These 'extremes in the spectrum of spatial, material and chemical disorganization' make recognition of the ideally well-organized elements of the structures difficult. However, after appropriate normalization of such tissues the 'feel' is quite different:

Poetry of Palpation

> You can feel the energy and tone flow into and through the myofascial unit....dissolving the 'glue' that, in holding the fascial envelopes together, has given the feeling of bunched and undifferentiated flesh.
> As fascial tone improves, individual muscles glide over one another, and the flesh – no longer 'too, too solid' – reminds the searching fingers of layers of silk that glide on one another with a suggestion of opulence.

Rolf's excitement is not feigned, Palpation of the body should change with practice from being a purely mechanical act into a truly touching and moving experience, in all senses of those words. Paul Van B. Allen D.O. pinpointed the need for concentrated application to the task of heightening ones perceptive (and therapeutic) skills:

> Let us lay down a few principles to guide us in the development of manual skills....It is commonplace to accept the need for basic principles and for practice, in developing manual skill to strike a golf ball, or a baseball, to roll a bowling ball, to strike a piano key or to draw a bow across strings, but we seldom, if ever anymore, think of manual skills in osteopathic practice in this way. Is it possible that osteopathic manipulation began to lose its effectiveness and to fall into disrepute even among our own people, when students no longer practiced to see through how many pages of *Gray's Anatomy* they could feel a hair?

> *(Academy of Applied Osteopathy Yearbook, 1964)*

(This was a written at a traumatic time for osteopathy in the United

States, when 2,000 Californian osteopaths gave up their D.O. status and accepted M.D. status in return for the turning of osteopathic colleges into medical schools. A resurgence of basic osteopathic teaching and skills has since reversed that catastrophe.)

All therapists who use their hands can ask themselves if they spend enough time refining and heightening their degree of palpatory sensitivity. The answer in many cases will be no, and hopefully this text will encourage a return to exercises such as this useful application of *Gray's Anatomy* (a telephone directory was used for this purpose in the author's training; it is equally effective).

Going beyond his despair at the loss of interest in palpatory skills, Allen makes another useful contribution:

> We will understand better what we feel if we attempt to describe it. In describing what is experienced through palpation we try to classify the characteristics of tissue states, thus not only clarifying our own observations but broadening our collective experience by affording a better means of communication between us and discussing (osteopathic) theory and method. We are accustomed to describing crude differences in what we feel by touch, the roughness of the bark of a tree or of a tweed coat, the smoothness of a glass or silk. We must now develop a language of nuances and I shall suggest only a few words from many to apply to palpable tissue states in an effort to describe them accurately.

Allen then launches into detailed descriptions of the meanings, as he sees them, of words such as 'density', 'turgidity', 'compressibility', 'tensile state (or response to stretch)' and 'elasticity'. His choice of words may not suit all but his idea is sound. We need to unleash a torrent of descriptive words for what we feel when we palpate and the text of the chapters covering various approaches to this most vital of procedures will hopefully inspire the reader to follow Allen's advice, to obtain a thesaurus and to look up as many words as possible accurately to describe the subtle variations in what is being palpated.

Viola Frymann reminds us that Dr Sutherland used the analogy of a bird alighting on a twig and then taking hold of it, when he tried to teach his students how to palpate the cranium. Some of the exercises in this book are derived from Frymann's work, and in many of these she echoes the ideas of Dr Van B. Allan that the student of palpation also practise the art of describing what they are feeling, either verbally or in writing. Dr Frymann's words can hopefully serve as a guide throughout this text:

> It is one thing to understand intellectually that physiological functions operate, and what may happen if they became disorganized. It is quite another thing, however to be able to place the hands on a patient and analyse the nature and the extent of the disorganization and know what can be done to restore it to normal, unimpeded, rhythmic physiology. This then is the task before us; to know what has happened and is happening to the tissues under our hands, and then to know what can be done about it and be able to carry it through.

Special Note
The Dominant Eye

Many osteopathic and chiropractic texts advise that, before
starting to palpate, you identify your dominant eye. Almost all of
us have one, and the reasoning is that you should position yourself
in relation to the patient, or body part, so that the dominant eye
has the clearest possible view of what is being observed. Clearly this
is of little importance if palpation with the eyes closed (a common
recommendation) is being employed. There will, however, be many
instances when visual impressions need to be combined with
palpation, for example in use of the 'red reaction', (see p. 34ff.).

- Make a circle with your first finger and thumb and, holding
  the arm out in front of your face, observe an object across
  the room, through that circle, with both eyes open.
- Close one eye. If the object is still in the circle, you now have
  your dominant eye open.
- If, however, the image shifts out of the circle when only one
  eye is open, open the closed eye and close the open eye, and
  the image should shift back into clear view, inside the circle.
- Thus the eye which sees the same view as you saw when both
  eyes were open is the one to use in close observation of the
  body.

If the patient is on an examination couch, you should approach the
couch from the side which will allow your dominant eye to be
closest to the centre of the couch. In some instances, when
symmetrical motion is being observed, such as when rib function is
being assessed, it is a mistake to closely observe one side and then
the other. You should instead rely on the sensitive discrimination
which peripheral vision offers. Focus on a point between the two
moving ribs and allow your peripheral vision to judge variations in
motion as the patient breathes. (If you are right-handed, with a
dominant left eye, or left-handed with a dominant right eye (both
are unusual combinations) you would probably make an excellent
batsman in cricket, or hitter in baseball.)

Chapter 2

First Steps in Skill Enhancement

The human hand is equipped with instruments to perceive changes in temperature, surface texture, surface humidity, to penetrate and detect successively deeper tissue textures, turgescence, elasticity and irritability. The human hand, furthermore, is designed to detect minute motion, motion which can only be detected by the most sensitive electronic pick-up devices available. This carries the art of palpation beyond the various modalities of touch into the realm of proprioception, of changes in position and tension within our own muscular system.

Viola Frymann's words define succinctly and with feeling, the tool we use and the task we perform when we palpate.

Different parts of the human hand are more or less able to discriminate variations in tissue features, such as relative tension, texture, degree of moisture, temperature and so on. This highlights the fact that any individual's overall palpatory sensitivity depends on a combination of different perceptive (and proprioceptive) qualities and abilities. These include the ability to register temperature variations and the subtle differences which exist in a spectrum of tissue states, ranging from very soft to extremely hard, as well as the ability to register the existence and size of extremely small entities such as are found in fibrotic tissue or trigger point activity, along with the sensitivity to distinguish between many textures and ranges in tone, from flaccid to spastic, and all the variables in between.

Professor Irvin Korr helps us to understand just why the hand is so delicately able to perform its many tasks:

Where do we find the greatest number of muscle spindles? Exactly where they logically belong. If the muscle spindle has to do with finely-tuned muscle activity, with measuring gains in extremely small lengths of muscle fibers, one would expect that for more complex movement patterns, as in the muscles of the hand, we would have a very large number of muscle spindles. And this is exactly what we find. The number of spindles per gram of muscle is only $1\frac{1}{2}$ in the latissimus dorsi; in the hand the number is close to 26. Functionally this of great significance.

(*Physiological Basis of Osteopathic Medicine*)

Physiology of Touch Some differences in palpatory ability result from variations in the number and type of sensory skin receptors in various anatomical regions, since this greatly influences the discriminatory capabilities of those regions. Light touch is generally accepted to be achieved via mechano-receptors such as Meissner's corpuscle, and Merkel's disk, as well as hair-root plexi, lying in the skin, muscles, joints and organs. They respond to mechanical deformation resulting from pressure, stretch or hair movement. It is in the skin that the greatest number of these receptors are found. Cruder touch perception is thought to relate to Krause's end-bulb, Ruffini's ending and Pacinian corpuscles.

Mechanoreceptors
Light touch:
    Meissner's corpuscle
    Merkel's disk
    Hair root plexus
Deep pressure:
    Pacininan corpuscle
Crude touch:
    Thought to be Krauses's endbulb
    Thought to be Ruffini's ending

Proprioception
Muscle length, tendon and limb position:
    Muscle spindle
    Golgi tendon organ
    Joint/kinesthetic receptors

Nociceptors
Pain:
    Free nerve endings

Thermoreceptors
Warmth:
    Thought to be free nerve endings
Cold:
    Thought to be free nerve endings
Internal temperature:
    Hypothalamic thermostat

Sensations of heat and cold are detected by thermo-receptors which are considered to be the free nerve endings in the skin. If cold is intense, detection is by nociceptors – specialized pain detectors – which are also free nerve endings. Primary (afferent) sensory neurons link the target organ (in this case skin) with the spinal cord or brain stem. Sensory units of this type serve an area of skin called a receptive field. These fields may overlap – if there are many sensory units crowded close together – and any tactile stimulation of such units (where there is close proximity and some degree of overlap) automatically results in signal transmission from neighbouring units to the Central Nervous System (CNS) being suppressed via inhibition of their synapses. This is known as lateral inhibition, and serves to sharpen perception of contrasts in whatever is being touched.

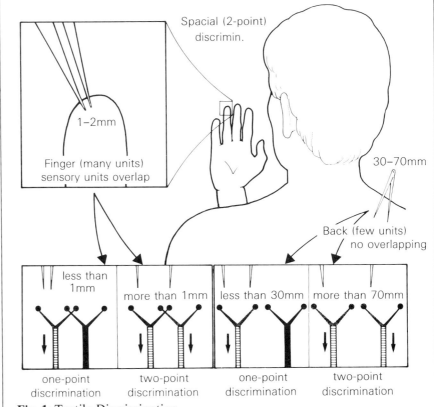

Fig. 1: Tactile Discrimination

Spacial discrimination: In the two-point test, the spacial discriminative ability of the skin is determined by measuring the minimum separable distance between two tactile point stimuli. The back of the hands, the back and legs rate low (50-100mm). The fingertips, lips and tongue rate high in this ability (1-3mm).

Intensity discrimination: Sensitive areas are also better able to discriminate differences in the intensity of tactile stimuli. Therefore, an indentation of 6 microns on the fingertip is sufficient to extract a sensation. This threshold is 4 times higher in the palm.

The degree of tactile sensitivity in any area is in direct proportion to the number of sensory units present and active in that area, as well as to the degree of overlap of their receptive fields, which vary in size. Small receptive fields with many sensory units therefore have the highest degree of discriminatory sensitivity. This can be assessed by use of what is called a two-point discrimination test; two sharp points are touched to the area, with the distance between them being varied until the shortest distance at which it is still possible to note that two and not one point is being touched is reached.

Measurement of the minimum separable distance between two tactile points of stimulus proves that the greatest degree of spatial discrimination exists on the surface of the tongue, the lips and fingertips (1–3 mm). In contrast, the back of the hands, the back and the legs have a poor degree of sensitivity (50 mm–100 mm).

Not only is there a difference of perception relating to spatial accuracy, but also one relating to intensity. An indentation of 6 microns is capable of being registered on the fingertips, while 24 microns of pressure is needed before the sensors in the palm of the hand reach their threshold and perceive the stimulus. The threshold on the backs of the hands, trunk and legs is some ten to twenty times higher than the fingertips, which, along the tongue, are the most sensitive palpatory units available to us.

It is unlikely that any clinical value can be attached to the tongue's capabilities, and so the remarkable discriminatory abilities of the fingertips are best used for our enhanced literacy in palpation. This is the majority viewpoint – some prominent dissenters hold that proprioceptive capabilities can be harnessed to a whole-hand contact, making this the more useful contact. This will be discussed further on p.20. Relatively weak stimulus to the fingertips can produce brain-cell activation and it is this brain–hand link which holds the key to palpatory literacy.

Variations in sensitivity – relating to both spatial and intensity factors – highlights the marked degree of variation between individuals. This may be because of anatomical differences, such as the number of receptors per square centimetre, a variation which would clearly alter the degree of perception possible. In any comparative study of human (or animal) anatomy there are clear and marked variations in size, number and position of almost all structures, not excluding neural receptors. Physiological differences also abound in any such examination and so it is a truism to note that not everyone will have the same degree of sensitivity when they palpate. Some will find it easy to perceive delicate pulsating rhythms, whereas others may have to work long and hard to heighten their sensibilities to the point where they can do so.

Receptor Adapt

Anatomical differences are not the only factors involved in variations in palpatory sensitivity; we have to try to overcome, by constant effort, a physiological response which 'switches off' (or decreases) the rate of firing of receptors when some stimuli are maintained. This relates to the activity of certain receptors, termed 'rapidly firing receptors', which tend to lose their sensitivity on any sustained contact. The receptors related to fine touch and pressure are of just this rapidly adapting type. Under normal conditions this is thought to have value in preventing our constant awareness of whatever is touching our body (clothing, for example) but it has a nuisance value for anyone attempting to palpate for any length of time.

By constrast mechano-receptors, serving joint and muscle, are slow adaptors, as are pain receptors. It is use of the proprioceptive receptors which some experts such as John Upledger suggest should be incorporated into the palpatory exercise, and their slow adaptation certainly adds weight to this suggestion. The alterations in sensitivity resulting from rapid adaptation to light touch is something which can be modified by practice, and the exercises which follow later in this chapter will help in this objective.

It is the *tips of the fingers or thumbs* which have the greatest discriminatory ability to measure variations in whatever is being felt. The skin surface itself, with its range of variations from hot or warm to cool or cold; thick or thin, dry, oily or moist; puffy or firm; smooth or rough and so on, is best assessed with the *pads of the fingers or the palm*, as a rule; the *dorsum of the hand* because of its sensitivity, is thought by some to be best for measuring the skin surface for temperature and moistness variations. (Mitchell seems to question this assumption, which he says is based mainly on histological data, suggesting that definitive tests should be carried out in which individuals who have been trained to enhance their 'temperature literacy' would have different parts of their hands assessed for sensitivity.)

Assessment of the depth of structures from the surface, as well as their relative size, is usually best achieved by the *finger tips* and to some extent the *palms of the hands*. The *palms* and *finger tips* are also the most useful contact for perception of variations in the status of osseous structures, through skin, fat, fascia and muscle.

The *whole hand* including the *fingers* (and incorporating reference to the proprioceptors in the forearms and wrists) is an accurate measuring instrument; the hands can be moulded to the surface in the activity of 'listening' for subtle physiological motions, such as primary respiratory motion in cranial osteopathic terminology, or visceral motion when organ position and function is being assessed. Subtle variations in amplitude and direction of such of movement as well as frequency of cycles of activity can readily be assessed in this way with practice.

If palpation is going to move beyond a simple assessment of the obvious characteristics of the tissues themselves, the hands need to register movement, pulsations and minor tremors and rhythms, along with variations in all or any of these as they respond to the palpatory processes. The *palmer finger surfaces* are most efficient for the role of picking up very fine vibration. William Walton D.O. summarized this as follows:

> Most authorities agree on two points. One is that the pads of the fingers are the most sensitive portions of the hands available to diagnosis; that part of the pad just distal to the last interphalangeal articulation is the most sensitive. The second point is that the thumb and first two fingers are the best to use. Which of these fingers or what combinations of them to use vary with the area under consideration, and the operator's own personal preference.
>
> (*Journal of the American Osteopathic Association*, August 1971)

Dr John Upledger differs markedly in his suggestions as to the ideal palpatory tool:

Most of you have been taught to palpate or touch with your fingertips...we, however, would urge you to palpate with your whole hand, arm, stomach or whatever part of your body comes into contact with the patient's body. The idea is to 'meld' the palpating part of your body with the body you are examining. As this melding occurs, the palpating part of your body does what the patient's body is doing. It becomes synchronized. Once melding and synchronization have occurred, use your own proprioceptors to determine what the palpating part of your own body is doing. Your proprioceptors are those sensory receptors located in the muscles, tendons, and fascia that tell you where the parts of your body are without using your eyes.

Upledger's ideas will be expanded on and some of his exercises for enhancement of palpatory skills examined as we progress.

Clyde Ford D.C. reminds us (*Where Healing Waters Meet*, Station Hill Press, New York 1989) that we commonly 'project' our sense of touch, giving the example of writing with a pencil. We feel the texture of the page, on which we are writing not at our skin surface or in our fingertips, but at the end of the pencil, thus demonstrating how our proprioceptive awareness can be projected.

He suggests you experiment by 'changing the pressure with which you grasp the pencil – you'll quickly discover that you can't write. The pressure exerted to hold the pencil needs to be constant so you can extend your perception to (the) pencil tip and thereby control the complex task of writing. A good craftsperson knows this instinctively. The woodworker's sense of touch extends to the teeth of the saw, a machinest's to the end of a wrench, a surgeon's to the edge of a scalpel, an artist's to the tip of a brush.'

In days gone by, when a physician had to diagnose by touch: 'A good practitioner did not feel a tumour at his fingertips but he projected his vibratory and pressure sensations into the patient.' So we regularly project our sense of touch beyond our physical being and, in palpation, says Ford, 'We merely make the ordinarily unconscious process available to our conscious mind.'

In so doing we 'cross the delicate boundary between self and other, to explore, to learn and ultimately to help.'

Mitchell, Moran and Pruzo, in their classic text *An Evaluation of Osteopathic Muscle Energy Procedure* explain what they believe palpation to be aiming at: 'Palpation is the art of feeling tissues with your hands in such a manner that changes in tension and position within these tissues can be readily noticed, diagnosed and treated.' This is the very simplest aim of palpation, for the method and the instrument (finger pads? whole hand?) it seems can vary, and the objectives can become every more refined. Mitchell, writing alone this time (*Journal of the American Osteopathic Association*, June 1976) examined the subject of the training and measurement of sensory literacy (he coupled visual and palpatory literacy into 'sensory literacy') in a wider sense:

> The necessity for projecting one's tactile senses to varying distances through an intervening medium must seem mystical and esoteric to many beginning

students. The projection of the palpatory sense through varying thicknesses of tissue is actually a refinement of the sense of tension and hardness. This sense is capable of even further refinement, through perceptual eidetic imagery, to be able to recognize, characterize, and quantify potential energies in living tissues. Thus some osteopaths are able to read in the tissues the exact history of past trauma.

Specific Objectives Coming back to more basic physical examination as it relates to superficial and then deep palpation, Walton points to specific objectives which should be looked for: 'There are five types of change to be noted by *superficial* palpation in both acute and chronic lesions: *skin changes, temperature changes, superficial muscle tensions, tenderness and oedema.*' And for *deeper palpation*: 'The operator increases the pressure on his palpating fingers sufficiently to make a contact with the tissues deep in the skin... six types of change may be noted: *mobility, tenderness, oedema, deep muscle tension, fibrosis and interosseous changes.* All but fibrosis can be perceived in both acute and chronic lesions.'

In order to achieve the basic objective of being able to assess and judge such changes, education of the hands and development of heightened proprioceptive sensibility in the detection and amplification of subtle messages is required (see exercise 14 p.27). This is then followed by appropriate interpretation of the information:

> *Detection* is a matter of being aware of the possible findings and practising the techniques required to expose these possibilities. *Amplification* requires localized concentration on a specific task and the ability to block out extraneous information. *Interpretation* is the ability to relate the information received via detection and amplification.

As indicated in Chapter 1, it is the detection and amplification aspects of palpation with which we are concerned, since what you subsequently do with any information thus gathered will largely depend upon your training and belief system.

Philip Greenman D.O. (*Principles of Manual Medicine*) defines the three stages of palpations as being Reception, Transmission and Interpretation. A useful warning is given that care be taken over the hands ('these sensitive diagnostic instruments') as we develop coordinated, symmetrical skills, linked with our visual sense:

Commonest Palpatory Mistake Avoidance of injury abuse is essential, hands should be clean, and nails an appropriate length. During the palpation the operator should be relaxed and comfortable to avoid extraneous interference with the transmission of the palpatory impulse. In order accurately to assess and interpret the palpatory findings it is essential that the physician concentrate on the act of palpation, the tissue being palpated, and the response of the palpating fingers and hands. All extraneous sensory stimuli should be reduced as much as possible. *Probably the most common mistake in palpation is the lack of concentration by the examiner* (My emphasis).

Moving beyond the physical assessments towards the palpation of subtle circulatory and energy rhythms and patterns, as described in craniosacral therapy, zero balancing and the work of various osteopathic researchers requires that palpation skills be further refined.

Where then should we begin in the process of developing and or enhancing our proprioceptive and palpatory skills? Exercises which can help in this task have been formulated by many experts, and a good starting point would be to practise the following until you are comfortable with your ability to obtain the information demanded without undue difficulty. These exercises are based on the advice and work of numerous individuals who have described specific methods for the acquisition of high levels of palpatory literacy. *These exercises are meant to be introduced more or less in sequence in order to gradually refine sensitivity*.

Important Descriptors

Before starting these exercises (which are not only useful for beginners but are excellent for refreshing the skills of the more experienced therapist) it is useful to prepare a number of comparative descriptive terms for that which will be palpated. Thus we should have a number of what Philip Greenman calls 'paired descriptors' (*Principles of Manual Medicine*). These can include superficial/deep, compressible/rigid, warm/cold, moist or damp/dry, painful/painfree, local or circumscribed/diffuse or widespread, relaxed/tense, hypertonic/hypotonic, normal/abnormal and so on.

It is also useful to begin when appropriate, to think in terms of whether any abnormality is acute, sub-acute or chronic. In making such an assessment it is useful to couple this with information from the patient in order to confirm the accuracy or otherwise of the finding. Thus if tissue feels chronically altered and the patient confirms that the area has been troublesome for longer than 4 weeks, an accurate 'reading' was made. In general terms acute conditions relate to the past few weeks; sub-acute to between 2 and 4 weeks, and chronic for longer than that. Obviously, in many instances, acute exacerbation of a chronic area may be what is being palpated, a confusing but useful palpatory exercise. The degree of change should also be noted, using a subjective scale for conditions which appear mild, moderate or severe. A simple numerical code can be used to identify where on this scale the palpated tissues lie.

Exercises

Viola Frymann summarized some very simple beginning points for developing sufficient sensitivity to commence efficient palpation. She advises, quite logically, that we palpate tissues direct, not through clothing, and that we remain as relaxed as possible during the whole process. This is important, as unnecessary tensions interfere with perception.

It is vital that we use only sufficient weight in our contact with the region being explored, and that this contact should be slowly applied to allow time for 'attunement' to the tissue being assessed:

The gauging of tissue resistance is attained by the application of your muscle sense, your work sense. It is not merely a contact sense, a touch sense, but sensations mainly derived from work being done by the muscles. This is what is meant by proprioception.

Some of Frymann's exercises will increase the sensitivity required for very light palpation needed for noting elasticity, turgor, moisture, sebaceous activity, relative warmth of coldness of tissues and so on.

Exercise 1. Sit at a table, wooden ideally, and while slowly and carefully palpating its upper surface with the eyes closed, try to locate the position of the legs. There will be less resilience – or greater resistance – to the palpating hand/fingerpads in areas where support lies under a particular part of the surface.

Exercise 2. Place a coin under a telephone directory and try to find it by careful palpation of the upper surface of the directory. If this is too difficult at first do it initially with a magazine, gradually increasing the thickness of the barrier between your fingers and the coin until the telephone directory presents no problem.

Exercise 3. Place a human hair under a page of a telephone directory and palpate for it through the page, eyes closed. Once this becomes relatively easy, place the hair under 2 pages and then 3, doing the same thing, feeling slowly and carefully for the slightly raised surface overlaying the hair. Now how long does it take you to feel the hair? Repeat until it is easy and quick.

Exercise 4. Sit at a table (blindfolded) and try to distinguish variations between objects made out of different materials: wood, plastic, metal, bone and clay for example. Describe what is being felt in terms of properties such as temperature, shape, surface texture, resilience, flexibility and so on. Do materials of organic and non-organic origin have a different feel? Can you differentiate between these and describe that difference?

Exercise 5. Van Allen developed a training method for enhancing perception of what he termed tissue 'density'. He obtained several blocks of wood, $2 \times 4 \times 18$ inches of very soft wood (pine) and of progressively harder woods (cherry, walnut, maple). He states:

Sliding one's fingers over these blocks revealed the differences in density and was a good exercise in developing tactile sensitivity. In some of these blocks I bored 3/4 inch holes from the underside, half the length, to within a quarter of an inch of the upper surface, and poured the holes full of lead, peaning it solidly with a ball-pean hammer. The blocks appeared uniform as they lay face up, with the leaded ends, some one way and some another. It was not too hard for most observers to tell which end was which as they slid their fingers over them. Osteopathic physicians varied widely in their ability to do this, some detecting the differences in one sweep of the fingers, others requiring many trials.

Those that did better in the 'test' were the practitioners known for their palpatory skills. Reproducing Van Allen's blocks, lead and all, may be somewhat difficult, but obtaining blocks of wood of uniform size but of differing density should not be difficult; schools could have an array of these for their students to palpate and assess.

Exercise 6. Mitchell suggests different ways of performing this sort of early exercise. He urges paired students to place objects (unseen by the student to be tested) in a box (or bag) with an opening through which the palpating student would reach to palpate. Mitchell suggests that such a 'black box' can be used as the first stage of learning to assess temperature, texture, thickness, humidity, tension or hardness, shape (stereognosis), position, proprioception, size, motion proprioception and so on.

Exercise 7. An elaboration on the use of a 'black box' which Mitchell discusses would be to enhance discriminatory faculties by including a variety of materials made of rubber, plastic, wood, metal and so on of varying thicknesses in the box. These would be evaluated and quantified with the results being discussed. These materials could contain another variation in which a rough textured material, say sandpaper of different degrees of roughness, could be covered by varying thicknesses of foam. In this way multiple variations could be created for the tuning of palpatory skills: 'Layers of materials of varying tension and hardness could be superimposed. For example, somatic soft tissues overlaying bone could be simulated with stratified layers of foam padding, sheet rubber, and vinyl fabric.'

In this way a training device with variable tensions could be constructed, says Mitchell, simulating muscular spasm, fibrotic changes, oedema and bony structures felt through varying thicknesses of soft tissue: 'It would be reasonable to expect that training with such devices would increase a student's confidence in his/her ability to tell the difference between spastic muscle and bone, or between hypertrophied muscle and contracted muscle.'

Exercise 8. Frymann suggests that the next objective should be to move from tools to begin to increase the student's ability to study anatomy using the hand instead of the eye. She suggests that the student sit, with eyes closed or wearing a blindfold, while palpating one of the cranial bones or any other bone, real or plastic if you are unfamiliar with cranial structures. Articular structures should be felt for and described in some detail (ideally with someone else handing the bone to you, and with findings being spoken into a tape recorder for self-assessment later, when the object/bone can be studied with eyes open).

The bone should be named, sided and its particular features discussed. If you are new to cranial structures this is an excellent educational method for becoming familiar with their unique qualities. While palpating this bone you should be asking:

- What is the nature of this object, is it plastic or bone?
- What would be the difference in feel between plastic and bone?

Bone, albeit dead, has a slight compressive resilience which plastic never has; plastic cannot achieve the detail of sutural digitation which bone contains either. Careful fingering of the unseen object would establish its shape, and if anatomy is well enough understood it could then be named and sided. *The whole process of palpating is enhanced, suggests Frymann, if the arms are supported so that the hands and fingers are unaffected by the weight of the arms.* Spend between 5 and 7 minutes palpating in this way.

Exercise 9. Whichever bone is used (cranial or otherwise) initially this should be followed by a blindfolded palpation of the same bone in a live subject, with its contours, sutures (if cranial), resilience and observed (not initiated) motion, being felt for and described. When comparison is made with the live bone in this way similarities and differences should gradually become apparent. The differences between the dead and live bone should be described and defined – ideally into a tape recorder.

Obviously the living bone would not be palpated directly, but through superficial tissue. This requires that the palpation become discriminating (Frymann talks of the 'automatic selection device of our consciousness') filtering out information offered by soft tissues which overlay the bone being assessed. By applying the attention of the mind to what is being palpated (for not less than 5 minutes in the early stages) subtle awareness of motion inherent in the live bone's existence should also become apparent. If this is a cranial bone there are three rhythms which can be felt for – pulsation, respiration and a slower rhythmic motion – and it is possible to learn to gradually learn to focus on one or other of these at will. We will come to exercises which will improve such discrimination later (p.30–1, 109ff.).

Exercise 10. In order to begin to learn to study and analyse more subtle connections Frymann then suggests that the student of palpation feels for a rhythmic motion by placing one hand on a spinal segment, from which stems the neurological supply to an area which is simultaneously being palpated by the other hand. By patient focusing for some minutes – eyes closed – on what is being felt, she states, 'A fluid wave will eventually be established between the two hands.'

Exercise 11. Mitchell makes the somewhat bizarre suggestion that the blindfolded student should palpate a live arm and simultaneously that of a cadaver which had been warmed to body temperature. Assuming no cadavers are available he then urges that palpation be performed on normal tissues and those of individuals with pathology such as limb paralysis. Simultaneous palpation of normal and diseased tissues offers an educational opportunity which all should aim to experience. Describe the different 'feel' of hypertonicity and hypotonicity after palpating for several minutes.

Exercise 12. Frymann simplifies the initial palpation of living tissue compared with non-living, sparing us the task of finding a corpse.

She suggests that the student of palpation should sit at a table opposite a partner, one of whose arms rests on the table, flexor surface upwards. This arm should be totally relaxed. The student lays a hand onto that forearm with attention focused on what the palmer surface of the fingers are feeling, the other hand resting on the firm table surface. This is to provide a contrast reference as the living tissue is palpated, to help to distinguish a region in motion from one without motion. The elbows of the palpater should rest on the table so that no stress builds up in the arm or shoulders.

Eyes closed, the student should project all his/her concentration into what the fingers are feeling, attuning to the arm surface. Gradually, focus should be brought to the deeper tissues under the skin as well, and finally to the underlying bone. When structure has been well noted the function of the tissues should be considered. Feel for pulsations and rhythms, periodically varying the pressure of the hand. At this stage Frymann urges you to: 'Pay no attention to the structure of skin, or muscle, or bone. Wait until you become aware of *motion*: observe and describe that motion, its nature, its direction, its rhythm and amplitude, its consistency or its variation.' This entire palpatory exercise should take not less than 5 minutes.

Exercise 13. When you have palpated an arm (or thigh, or indeed any other part of the body) to the point where you are clearly picking up the sensations of motion and rhythmic pulsation, place your other hand on the other side of the same limb. Is this hand picking up the same motions? Are the sensations moving in the same direction, with the same rhythm and is there the same degree of amplitude to the motion as the first sensation?

In health they will be the same. When there is a difference it represents 'tissue memory' of trauma or some other form of dysfunction. Take 5 to 10 minutes to perform this exercise.

Exercise 14. Frymann suggests that on another occasion (or at the same session) you palpate one limb with one hand (upper arm) and another limb (thigh for example) with the other, and that you 'rest in stillness until you perceive the respective motions within'. Ask yourself whether the rhythms you are feeling are synchronous and moving in the same direction. Are they consistent or do they undergo cyclical changes, periodically returning to the starting rhythmic pattern?

You may actually sense, she says, that the force being felt seems to carry your hands to a point beyond the confines of the body, pulling in one direction more than another, with little or no tendency to return to a balanced neutral position. This may represent the energy from a traumatic incident which is still manifest in the tissues. Careful questioning will often confirm the nature and direction of a distant blow or injury.

As we will discover in Chapter 4, researchers such as Becker and Smith have mapped this territory well, and have given us strong guidelines as to how we may move towards understanding such phenomena; Frymann's exercise is a first step in that direction. Take 5 to 10 minutes to perform this assessment.

Exercise 15. Upledger suggests starting with the regular practising of assessments of more obvious pulsating rhythms, such as those in cardiovascular pulses. He describes the first stages of this learning process thus:

With the subject lying comfortably supine, palpate the radial pulses. Feel the obvious peak of the pulsation. Tune in also to the rise and fall of the pressure gradient.

How long is diastole?

What is the quality of the rise of pulse pressure after diastole?

Is it sharp, gradual, smooth?

How broad is the pressure peak?

Is the pressure descent rapid, gradual, smooth or stepped?

Memorize the feel of the subject's pulse so that you can reproduce it in your mind after you have broken actual physical contact with the subject's body. You can often sing a song after you have heard it a few times; similarly, you should be able to mentally reproduce your palpatory perception of the pulse after you have broken contact.

Upledger then suggests you do the same thing with the carotid pulse, and subsequently palpate both radial and carotid at the same time, and compare them. This should take around 3 to 5 minutes initially.

Note: There are some very important lessons to be learned in performing simple pulse-taking. Frymann analyses some of the almost instinctive strategies we adopt if we do this well, and which all should consider as they perform exercise 15.

a. If the patient has a relatively normal systolic pressure (120 mmHg), any digital pressure on the pulse will obliterate it.

b. If the pressure is very light, say only 10 mmHg, only a very faint sensation will be palpated, if anything at all.

c. If, however, a light initial pressure is *gradually* increased, a variety of pulsation sensations will be noted, until the pulse is obliterated when the digital pressure overcomes the blood pressure. Indeed, as Frymann notes, this is how blood pressure was assessed before the introduction of the sphygmomanometer.

The student of palpation should experiment with variation of the degree of pressure, noting the subtle differences which are then perceived. We are learning to control the degree of applied digital pressure so that we meet that demanded by particular tissues, in order to gain optimal access to the locked-in information. Frymann states:

The examiner must supply the equal and opposite force to that of the tissue to be studied. The pressure in the eyeball can be estimated by attaining a balance of pressure between the examining finger and the intraocular pressure. The maturity of an abcess can be estimated similarly. Action and reaction must be equal.

This is a vital lesson in learning palpation.

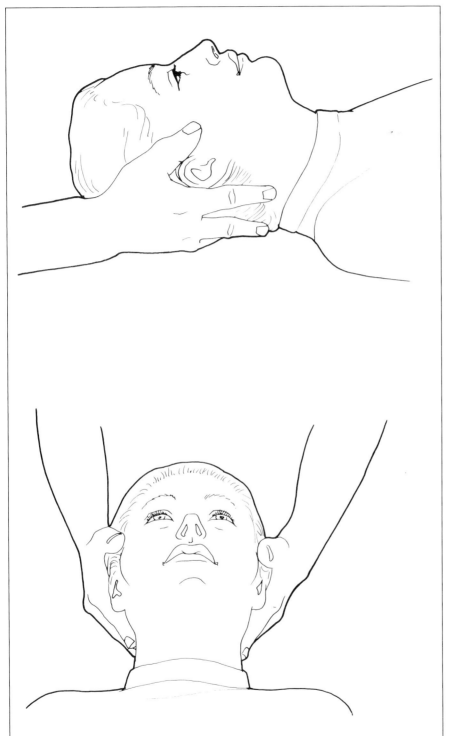

Fig. 2: Hand position for palpation of cardiovascular activity, inherent motion and other cranial rhythms.

Exercise 16. Next lay your hands on the upper thorax of the supine patient and palpate cardiovascular activity; focusing on the various characteristics of the perceived pulsations, alter your focus to the breathing pattern and its multiple motions. Practise switching attention from breathing to cardiovascular and back again until you are comfortable with the idea of screening out 'background' information from that which you want to examine. Spend 5 to 7 minutes doing this initially.

Exercise 17. Next rest the patient's head on your hands, with no more than a few grams of contact pressure from your whole hand/finger contact. The occiput should be resting on your palms and hypothenar region. Sitting with your eyes closed pay attention to cardiovascular activity (arterial pulsation, general pulsation in time with cardiac function and so on) as it is being sensed by these contacts.

After a while alter your focus, screening out cardiovascular activity, and see what you can feel in relation to cranial motion, coordinated with the breathing rhythm. Can you sense a very slight motion of the neck in time with respiration? Describe this after 3 to 5 minutes of palpation.

Exercise 18. Next screen out both the cardiovascular and the respiratory motions and see what else you can feel. Imagine your hands are totally linked to the head, without more than a few grams of pressure, and with this whole hand contact shift your focus to the proprioceptors in your wrist and lower arm. Sense what these are feeling. Magnify in this way the very small amount of actual motion available for palpation and you should gradually begin to feel as though quite a considerable degree of motion is taking place, as though the entire head were expanding and contracting laterally to a very slow rhythm, unrelated to cardiovascular or respiratory function, about 6 to 12 times per minute. Trust what you feel uncritically at this stage. Can you sense this rhythm? Take 5 to 7 minutes to do this carefully.

Exercise 19. Next, can you also sense a very slight dipping forward of the occiput as this expansion occurs under your hands, with a return to neutral as the head 'narrows'?

Can you, through the available contact of your middle and ring fingers, sense what is happening at the same time to the temporal or mastoid area?
Describe this.

Can you, through your thumb contact, sense what the parietal bones are doing as these rhythmic pulsations occur? Describe this.

We will return to Upledger's exercises in a later section where we will examine palpation of craniosacral rhythms throughout the body, and assess your initial 'findings' and descriptions. Spend not less than 5 minutes assessing these various motions.

Exercise 20. Have the partner/patient supine. The student of palpation slides his/her dominant hand beneath the sacrum so that the finger-tips rest at the base of the sacrum spreading from one sacro-iliac articulation to the other. The coccyx should be gently cradled in the heel of the hand and the forearm and elbow resting comfortably on the surface of the treatment table. The student can kneel or sit in order that he/she is as comfortable as possible during the 10 minutes or so of this exercise.

With eyes closed, all sensations reaching the palpating hand should be focused on. Is there any palpable rhythm synchronous with normal respiration? If so ask the patient to hold their breath, and observe what happens to the sacral motion. Is there still a subtle motion palpable as the breath is held?

As respiration resumes feel how this subtle motion alters again. It should be possible gradually to learn to screen the motion related to breathing from the more subtle 'cranial respiratory' rhythm. Spend as long as possible studying these subtle variations in sacral motion.

Note: (The ability to know what normal tissue feels like is a most useful palpatory exercise, since anything which feels other than normal is bound to be evidence of dysfunction. This suggests that it is useful to perform such exercises with people who are relatively young and 'normal', before finding individuals who are older, or who have suffered injury or stress in the tissues you intend palpating).

Philip Greenman (*Principles of Manual Medicine*) describes some excellent exercises – for both beginners and the more experienced – to increase palpation skills. These have been summarized as follows:

Exercise 21. Sit, with someone else, facing each other across a narrow table. You are going to examine each other's left forearms with your right hands, so place the left forearms on the table, palm downwards and rest the right (palpating) hand and fingers on your partners left forearm as they rest theirs on your forearm, just below the elbow.

The initial evaluation, without movement, calls for the mind to focus on what is being left. How warm/cool, dry/moist, thick/thin, rough/smooth is the palpated skin?

You and your partner should now turn the forearm over so that the same questions can be answered regarding the volar surface. Compare what was palpated on the dorsal surface with what was palpated on the volar surface. Evaluate and put words to the differences noted in texture, temperature, thickness and so on.

Exercise 22. In the same position, make small hand motions while a firm contact is being maintained with the skin, moving this in relation to its underlying tissues. Move the hand both longitudinally and horizontally, in relation to the forearm, and evaluate what is being palpated as to the subcutaneous fascial tissues. Try to assess its thickness and elasticity. Compare the findings from the dorsal and volar surfaces of your partners forearm.

Exercise 23. With this same contact palpate the subcutaneous fascial layer for the arteries and veins which lie in it. Identify and describe what you feel. Use an anatomical atlas if you are rusty on this part of anatomy.

Exercise 24. In the same position, think of the deeper fascia and increase your hand pressure until this is sensed. Use slow horizontal movements of the hands/fingers and try to identify thickened areas of fascia which act as envelopes which compartmentalize and separate muscle bundles.

It is in the subcutaneous and deeper fascial layers that much somatic dysfunction is found, ranging from trigger points to stress bands relating to overuse, misuse or abuse.

Exercise 25. With the same position and contact feel through the fascia to the muscle fibres and see whether you can feel their direction of action. You and your partner should now slowly open and close the left fist in order order to tense and relax the muscles being palpated. Sense the variations in the muscle fibres as this takes place.

Next you should both hold your left fists closed, strongly, as you palpate the hypertonic state of the forearm muscles, a most useful preparation for what will be palpated in most patients where overuse, misuse or abuse has been operating. Describe the textures and variations in tone which you have noted during this exercise.

Exercise 26. With the arm being palpated now relaxed, move your palpating fingers down the forearm and identify the interface between muscle and tendon (musculotendinous junction); continue to palpate the tendon itself on towards its point of insertion, where the tendon is bound to the wrist by a structure which overlays it, the transverse carpal ligament. Palpate this and see whether you can identify the various directions of fibre angle.
Which way does the tendon run?
Which way does the ligamentous structure run?
Describe their characteristics and 'feel'.

Exercise 27. Move back up to the elbow and with your middle finger resting in the hollow on the dorsal side of the elbow and your thumb on the ventral surface of the elbow, palpate the radial head.

Feel its shape and texture. How hard is it? Does it move on slight pressure? What do you feel if you move your finger and thumb slightly higher on the elbow, over the joint space itself?

You should not be able to feel the joint capsule unless there exists gross pathology of the joint. With the contact here you are just above the joint. Have your partner slowly actively pronate and supinate the arm, and see what you feel between finger and thumb.
How does the end of range of motion vary with the action of pronation and supination?
Is it symmetrical?
Describe the end-feel. (See p.151).

Which end of range seems firmer/tighter (which has the harder end-feel) supination or pronation?

Exercise 28. Now use your left hand to hold the hand and wrist of the arm you are palpating with your right hand. Introduce passive supination and pronation as you palpate the radiohumeral joint. Assess the total range of motion as you slowly perform these movements. You are receiving two sets of proprioceptive information at this stage, from the palpating hand and the one which is introducing motion.

Describe the range and the end-feel, in both supination and pronation when these are passively introduced, as well as comparing active with passive findings.

Does supination or pronation have the harder or softer end-feel, and which seems to have the greatest range of motion?

Are you aware of the build-up of tension as you approach the end of the range of movement?

Are you equally aware of the sense of tissue freedom as you move away from that barrier?

Try to become aware of changes, which can be called 'ease' and 'bind', as you move the joint in varying directions.

Can you find a point of balance somewhere between the ends of range of motion in pronation and supination, where tissues feel at their most free? If so you have found what is called the physiological neutral point, or point of balance, which is a key feature of functional osteopathic treatment. We will be returning to this concept, and will perform more exercises involving the neutral point in later chapters (notably Chapter 7).

Dr Greenman cautions that the most common errors in the application of these palpation exercises (and all palpation) are a lack of concentration, the use of excessive pressure, and too much movement. In other words, go lightly and slowly, and above all focus on what you are feeling if you want to palpate effectively.

These first exercises will help to grant the student of palpation an initial ability to differentiate (and describe) the shape, size, texture, flexibility and temperature of varying thicknesses and combinations of a variety of inorganic materials; to be able to discriminate between organic and inorganic materials, living and dead materials and tissues, living tissues of varying states of health, and the first stages of assessment of body pulsations and rhythms, with the facility to screen one from another at will being a key stage in palpatory literacy. It may also be possible to sense the forces associated with 'tissue memory' which will be examined more closely in later chapters.

All these exercises can be varied and altered to meet particular needs, they represent the ideas of some of the leading experts in the field and provide a starting point in the adventure in exploration of inner space which will follow.

We will now focus on palpation of the skin itself.

Red, White and Black Reaction

A number of researchers and clinicians have described an assortment of responses in the form of 'lines', variously coloured from red to white and even blue-black, after application of local skin dragging, with a finger or probe. Carl McConnell D.O., in his classic text *The Practice of Osteopathy* published in 1899, states:

> I begin at the first dorsal and examine the spinal column down to the sacrum by placing my middle fingers over the spinous processes and standing directly back of the patient draw the flat surfaces of these two fingers over the spinous processes from the upper dorsal to the sacrum in such a manner that the spines of the vertebrae pass tightly between the two fingers; thus leaving a red streak where the cutaneous vessels press upon the spines of the vertebrae. In this manner slight deviations of the vertebrae laterally can be told with the greatest accuracy by observing the red line. When a vertebra or section of vertebrae are too posterior a heavy red streak is noticed and when a vertebra or section of vertebrae are too anterior the streak is not so noticeable.

A little more recently, Marshall Hoag D.O., in *Osteopathic Medicine*, regarding examination of the spinal area writes:

> With firm but moderate pressure the pads of the fingers are repeatedly rubbed over the surface of the skin, preferably with extensive longitudinal strokes along the paraspinal area. The blunt end of an instrument or of a pen may be used to apply friction, since the purpose is simply to detect colour change, but care must be taken to avoid abrading the skin. The appearance of less intense and rapidly fading colour in certain areas as compared with the general reaction is ascribed to increased vasoconstriction in that area, indicating a disturbance in autonomic reflex activity. The significance of this red reaction and other evidence of altered reflex activity in relation to (osteopathic) lesions has been examined in research. Others give significance to an increased degree of erythema or a prolonged lingering of the red line response.

John Upledger writes of this phenomenon:

> Skin texture changes produced by a facilitated segment are also palpable as you lightly drag your fingers over the nearby paravertebral

area of the back. I usually do skin drag evaluations moving from the top of the neck to the sacral area in one motion. Where your fingertips drag on the skin, you will probably find the facilitated segment. After several repetitions, with increased force, the affected area will appear redder than nearby areas. This is the 'red reflex'.

Muscles and connective tissue at this level will

1. have a 'shoddy' feel (like BB's under the skin);
2. be more tender to palpation;
3. be tight and tend to restrict vertebral motion; and
4. exhibit tenderness of the spinous processes when tapped by fingers or a rubber hammer (*Craniosacral Therapy*).

Roger Newman Turner N.D., D.O., in his book *Naturopathic Medicine* describes the research of another osteopath/naturopath, Keith Lamont N.D., D.O., who first described the 'black line' phenomenon:

It is a common observation of osteopaths who use a spinal meter, to detect the most active lesions, that pressure on either side of the spine with a hemispherical probe of approximately 0.5 cm diameter, will, in some patients, illicit a dark blue or black line. The pressure of the probe is usually very light since it is intended to register variations in skin resistance, but it has a pinching-off effect on the arterioles and venules of the capillary network beneath the skin. Local engorgement of the capillary bed with deoxygenated venous blood causes the appearance of the line which slowly fades as the circulation returns.

This is considered to relate to a nutrient deficit in those patients in whom this sign is seen:

Keith Lamont, who first drew attention to the Black Line Phenomenon, has found that administration of vitamin E, bioflavonoid complex and homoeopathic ferum phosphate will correct this deficiency.

Bertrand DeJarnette D.C. the developer of sacrocranial technique, writes extensively on the subject of the 'red reaction', with some complex interpretations suggested (*Reflex Pain*, 1934). DeJarnette initially makes assessments of patients (partly based on blood pressure readings) into various categories, during which process he has them treated in order to alter the relative oxygenation levels which are assumed on the basis of these categories. None of these methods are pertinent to this survey of skin reactions, but are a necessary preamble to his descriptions, which would be confusing otherwise. In a type 1 patient, who has received the appropriate preliminary attention as outlined ('carbon dioxide elimination technic'):

Sit or stand immediately behind the patient facing the patient's back. Have the patient bend slightly forward. Be sure the light is even on the patient's back to avoid shadows. Place the index and middle fingers of your right hand upon the 7th cervical vertebra, having the two fingers about an inch lateral from the spine of the 7th cervical vertebra. Keep the fingers evenly spaced as you go down the spine, so each line is as straight as possible. For the type 1 patient (normal BP after appropriate techniques) use a light touch. To produce an even pressure of both fingers on the back they may be fortified by placing the fingers of the left hand over them. As you go down the spine, your pressure will be just hard enough to cause the fingers to dent the skin.

Now draw your fingers down the spine very quickly ending at the coccyx. Step back and watch the reaction. A red line will usually appear all the way down the spine. This soon starts to fade and the fading is what you must watch. The area that appears Reddest *as this fading starts, is the major* [lesion] for this patient and should be marked with a skin pencil. You will often notice on this type of patient that the major area is much wider than any other area of your lines down the back. This is caused by tissue infiltration.

The type 2 patient will have slightly high blood pressure after DeJarnette's preliminary treatment. After adopting the same starting position:

Making a firm pressure, draw fingers down the spine, with a fairly slow motion. You should be able to count to 15 while drawing the fingers from the 7th cervical to the coccyx, by counting steadily. With a good light on the back, the results should show a line which becomes red, some portions brighter and some very faintly coloured. Now watch the lines fade. The area which shows the Whitest is marked as the major [lesions] for this is the most anaemic spinal muscle area. It will be paler than any portion of skin on the patient's body.

Moving next to the final category which interests us in this survey, (high blood pressure) DeJarnette asks that you adopt the same start position and then:

Making heavy pressure, come down the spine slowly, counting 20 as you go from 7th cervical to coccyx. Now watch the reaction. The line that shows the Whitest is the major [lesion]. In this type the blood pressure is over 180 (systolic) the whitest area shows a waxy, pale colour and may persist for several minutes.

Professor Irvin Korr, writing of his years of osteopathic research (*The Physiological Basis of Osteopathic Medicine*) described how this red reflex phenomenon was shown to correspond well with areas of lowered electrical resistance, which themselves correspond accurately to pain threshold patterns and areas of cutaneous and deep tenderness. However, he cautions:

You must not look for perfect correspondence between the skin resistance (or the red reflex) and the distribution of deeper pathologic disturbance, because an area of skin which is segmentally related to a particular muscle does not necessarily overlie that muscle. With the latissimus dorsi, for example, the myofascial disturbance might be over the hip but the reflex manifestations would be in much higher dermatomes because this muscle has its innervation from the cervical part of the cord.

By use of a mechanical instrument which quantified the pressure applied at a constant speed, and then measuring the duration of the redness after the frictional stimulator had passed over the skin, Korr could detect areas of intense vasocontriction which corresponded well with dysfunction elicted by manual clinical examination.

It could be said that the opportunity to 'feel' the tissues was being ignored during all these 'strokes', and 'drawing' of the fingers down the spinal musculature. This was not lost on Marsh Morrison D.C. who describes his views thus:

> Run your fingers longitudinally down alongside the dorsal and lumbar vertebrae (anywhere from the spinous processes extending laterally up to two inches) and stop at any spot of tissue which seems 'harder' or different from normal tissue. These thickened areas, stringy ligaments, bunched muscle bounds, all represent indurated tissue; they are usually protective and indicate irritation and dysfunction. Once these indurated areas are palpated press down and almost always they will be sensitive, indicating a need for treatment (*Lecture Notes*).

Morrison used a technique for easing such contractions similar to that later described by Lawrence Jones D.O. in his strain counterstrain system. (Morrison's and Jones' methods are described in my book *Soft Tissue Manipulation*).

Clearly there is a good deal to learn from the simple procedure of stroking the paraspinal muscles. Whether or not DeJarnette's preliminary methods are validated does not alter the possible wisdom of his subsequent observations, employing as it does variable pressures and looking at the process fading rather than the initial red reaction, for evidence of altered function. Similarly, Lamont's nutritional observations would need verification, something which does not alter the fact that some patients demonstrate this unusual 'black streak'. The simpler observations of Upledger, Hoag, Morrison and McConnell are readily applicable, and should be tested against known dysfunction to assess the usefulness of these methods during assessment.

Postscript: How do you know whether your palpating fingers or thumbs are applying equal pressure bilaterally during such assessments, or when palpating elsewhere, bilaterally (as in many exercises in Chapter 7)? A useful guide to the uniformity of pressure can be obtained by comparing the relative blanching of your nailbeds; are they equally white, pink, red?

Chapter 3

Palpating and Assessing the Skin

The significance of palpated changes in the skin may not always be clear, and yet this boundary which separates the individual from the outside world, is a vital potential source of information. Contact with someone else's skin rapidly breaks barriers and opens a relationship of unique privilege, something which is used to great advantage by 'bodyworkers' who focus on the mind as well as the physical condition of their patients. The body surface reflects the state of the mind intimately, altering its electrical as well as its palpable physical properties.

Deane Juhan, in his book *Job's Body* sets the scene for our understanding of the skin's importance:

> The skin is no more separated from the brain than the surface of a lake is separated from its depths; the two are different locations in a continuous medium. 'Peripheral' and 'central' are merely spatial distinctions, distinctions which do more harm than good if they lure us into forgetting that the brain is a single functional unit, from cortex to fingertips and toes. *To touch the surface is to stir the depths* (My italics).

Learning to read changes on this surface is not easy, but contact with it provides a chance for exploration of much that is obvious and much that is deeply hidden. We will examine various concepts which relate to the mind–body link in Chapter 10. At this stage we need to look more closely at some of the physical characteristics of the skin.

As mentioned in the previous chapters, the changes which should be easily read by the literate palpator include the relative degree of warmth/coolness, dryness/moisture, smoothness/roughness, elasticity/rigidity as well as the relative degree of thickness of the skin in the region. Much research and clinical experience suggests that altered skin physiology of this sort is often an end result of dysfunction involving the sympathetic nervous system, as it relates to the musculoskeletal system.

In order to understand some of the dynamics involved in skin function and dysfunction, as well as some of the potential pitfalls possible in skin palpation, a brief examination of some aspects of the physiology of skin is necessary. Credit for the main thrust of the material in this section should go to the research of a group of scientists working in the United States: Adams, Steinmetz, Heisey, Holmes and Greenman. Their review 'Physiologic basis for skin properties in palpatory physical diagnosis' (*Journal of American Osteopathic Association*, February 1982) is a clear examination of some of the main interacting elements which make the skin such a critical area in palpation.

The skin contains nearly 750,000 sensory perceptors which vary in the density of their presence in different regions, from 7 to 135 per square centimeter. However it is not neural endings which receive attention from these researchers, rather they focus much of their attention onto the characteristics of human skin which derive from the activities of atrichial sweat glands, the secretions of which, apart from playing a role in temperature control, influence 'the energy and mass transfer characteristics of skin as well as altering its properties by establishing different levels of epidermal hydration and salinization'.

They ask us to make a clear distinction between epitrichial and atrichial sweat glands, the former being associated with hair shafts and the latter emptying directly on the skin, and thus directly influencing the important areas of skin friction and heat transfer properties. Those atrichial glands on the palmer surface of the hand (and the soles of the feet) have only a small potential for influencing heat loss, but are important in being capable of modifying skin friction and pliability. It is of considerable clinical importance that the atrichial sweat glands are totally controlled by the sympathetic division of the autonomic nervous system, since this renders any palpable changes which sweat activity might produce capable of being influenced by reflex activity, such as occurs when trigger points are active and when emotional or stress factors are operating. The chemical mediator between the motor nerve and the secretory tubule of atrichial sweat glands is acetylcholine, a neurotransmitter which increases the tendency for muscles to contract.

The complexities of water movement through the skin need not concern us at this stage, apart from a need to emphasize that the mechanical, electrical and heat transfer properties and characteristics of the skin are altered by this process.

As sweating occurs liquid is not only passed through the tubule but diffuses laterally into surrounding peritubular drier skin areas. Even when there is no obvious sweat on the skin surface sweat gland activity in the underlying skin continues, with some of the water which spreads into surrounding skin being reabsorbed. This mechanism is compared with the way in which the kidney tubule deals with sugar in the urine:

> By the same logic that it is incorrect to deduce that there is no sugar in the renal glomerular filtrate because none is detected in the urine, it is similarly incorrect to conclude that the sweat glands are inactive because there is no water on the skin surface.

> (Adams, Steinmetz *et al*.)

Low-level sweat gland activity has the effect of altering the degree of skin friction. Friction is low when the skin is dry and higher as it becomes moist, decreasing again when sweating becomes very intense. It is hard to turn a page with a dry finger; moisten it slightly and the task is easier, but a very sweaty hand cannot grasp anything easily. We can conclude that there is a narrow range of epidermal water content that produces maximum frictional contact at the skin surface.

This knowledge may help us understand some of the reasons for the regional variations in skin friction ('skin drag') noted on palpation. Adams, Steinmetz, Heisey, Holmes and Greenman ask:

> Is this possible that regional differences in 'skin drag' perceived by the examining physician are related to segmentally active, autonomic reflexes that trigger chronic, low level, atrichial sweat gland activity, which in turn increases local epidermal hydration and skin friction at a defined body site? Do these reflexes produce, through chronic sweat gland activity, changes in the mechanical properties of the skin's surface, similar to those you might detect on the wrist skin surface when a watchband is initially removed?

(Initially when the skin under a watchstrap is stroked there will be a high level of epidermal water which will make the friction level high, with a great deal of skin drag. After a while this is lost and the degree of drag will be similar to the surrounding skin characteristics).

This insight into the pathophysiology of skin should help us to understand just why Dr Karel Lewit is able to identify trigger point activity (or any other active reflex activity) by assessing the degree of elasticity in the overlaying skin and comparing it with neighbouring tissue. He terms local skin areas of this type 'hyperalgesic skin zones'. It also explains why, prior to the introduction of methods of electrical detection of acupuncture points, any skilled acupuncturist could find the points very quickly indeed by palpation, and also why measurement of the electrical resistance of the skin can now do this even more quickly.

We will examine some of Lewit's thoughts and directions later in this chapter, but first we will see how the degree of epidermal hydration influences our perception of warmth or cold in the tissues being palpated, and how the condition of our own skin affects palpation.

Clyde W. Ford, in his study of palpation and subtle manipulation (*Where Healing Waters Meet*, Station Hill Press, New York 1989) has a quite different interpretation of the mechanics of 'skin drag', outlined on p.129.

Learning to Measure Skin Temperature by Touch

Exercise 1. As you sit reading this page, palpate several different materials in the room in which you are sitting. Palpate something made of wood, metal, plastic, china and paper. All these objects are in a room in which we can presume that the ambient temperature is uniform; were they measured with a thermocouple, they would show almost exactly the same reading. But there is a distinct difference in temperature as you feel them. Why is this?

Exercise 2. Stand barefoot on a cold tile, marble or plastic floor.

Rest one foot on the floor and the other on a rug or towel which has been in the room for some time. One foot feels cold, the other does not. And yet the temperature of the floor and the rug is almost certainly the same. Why the perceived difference; in relation to palpation, where does this leave us in terms of the accuracy of what we think we 'feel'?

The variables which influence heat flow from the object which we are feeling to the surface of the unit we are using to feel with (fingertips, hand) are related to the thermal properties of these two 'exchanging surfaces'. These thermal properties include:

- The surface areas of the exchanging surfaces
- The differences in temperature between the exchanging surfaces
- The distance over which heat is being transferred
- The intrinsic properties of heat conduction associated with the object being palpated and the palpatory unit.

This last factor needs some clarification. This characteristic is called the thermal conducting coefficient (TCC). The TCC of a tiled floor is greater than the rug, and this causes the thermoreceptors in the foot on the tiled floor to be more rapidly cooled than the other foot. Your perception of one foot being colder than the other is accurate, but it does not relate to any differences in the temperature of the surfaces on which you are standing.

> If it can be rationally assumed or independently verified that two objects that feel different in temperature are actually at the same temperature then the difference in responding thermoreceptors can be attributed to a difference in thermal conductivity (or some other heat transfer property) of the object(s) being examined, *but not to a difference in temperature.*

This is clearly of great significance when it comes to making clinical judgements as to how warm or cool an area of skin is.

The Effect of Hydration on Temperature Judgement
A further complication becomes apparent when we examine the influence of the degree of epidermal hydration in those palpated tissues (and in the palpating hand).

> **Exercise 3.** Take any two objects which you have previously palpated for temperature difference, say a pencil and a metal key. Once again palpate these by hand and sense the difference in thermal sensation reaching the thermoreceptors in your hand. Try this first with hands dry and then moisten the fingertips (or whatever part of the hand is being used to palpate for temperature difference).

> **Exercise 4.** Next try to see whether the supposed thermal sensitivity of the dorsal aspect of the hand is indeed greater than that noted by the palm or finger pad when assessing the wooden pencil and the metal key.

Exercise 5. Now test these same objects again, but this time use the tongue tip as your 'palpating' organ. Note how much more clearly you can sense the apparent differences in temperature.

The thermoreceptors in the palmer surface are far more densely sited than on the dorsum of the hand, and are even more closely packed on the tip of the tongue (where they are close to the surface), making these regions more sensitive for palpation of heat. This means that despite the differences in epidermal thickness on the dorsum of the hand as compared with the palmer surface, the palm is usually a better place to make contact when seeking thermal information.

Also note that the relative dampness or otherwise of the palpating surface influences perception of heat. This is because of better conduction when water is present; the temperature of the thermoreceptors is closer to that of the object being examined than it would be with a dry contact.

We need to remain aware of the fact that our own state of hydration, our peripheral circulatory efficiency, our sympathetic nervous system activity, and a number of other variables, including ambient humidity and temperature, will influence thermal perception as we palpate. Adams and his colleagues summarize the problem of understanding the variables:

The thermoreceptors in an examining finger are part of a complex heat exchange system. The temperature that is felt by the examiner is directly related to the rate of action potential formation on afferent, sensory nerves arising from thermoreceptors near the dermo-epidermal junction. Their temperature is strongly dependent on heat brought to the skin (or taken away from it) by the circulating blood.

The perceived temperature is also determined by the rate of heat transfer out of, or into, the examiner's skin from the patient's skin, which relates to such factors as the area of contact, thickness of skin in both examiner and patient, and the status of epidermal hydration in both, as well as heat transfer characteristics (which will be influenced by factors such as material trapped between the two skin surfaces [examiner and patient] including air, water, lotion, grease or oil, dirt, fabric and so on). All or any of these variables will be operating each time we palpate, and to some extent at least, their net effect needs to be taken into consideration.

Exercise 6. Slowly and carefully, palpate the back or abdomen for temperature variations of the skin:
a. When the subject has been lying still for some minutes in a room of normal temperature/humidity.
b. When the subject has actively skipped, jogged, danced or performed some other exercise for some minutes.
c. When you have performed similar exercise for some minutes.
Are there any differences noted between a, b and c?
Vary your contact so that sometimes you use the palmer and

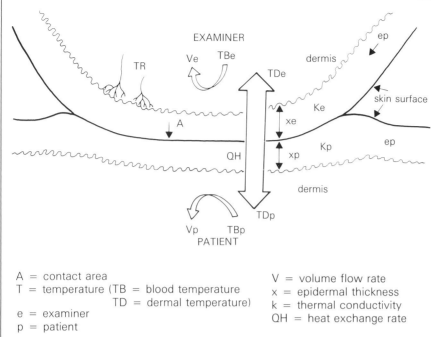

A = contact area
T = temperature (TB = blood temperature
                 TD = dermal temperature)
e = examiner
p = patient

V = volume flow rate
x = epidermal thickness
k = thermal conductivity
QH = heat exchange rate

Fig. 3: This diagram depicts some of the physical and physiologic factors that affect the thermoreceptor (TR) discharge rate and consequently the temperature sensed in an examiner's skin in contact with a patient's skin. The temperature and its rate of change of the examiner's thermoreceptors are functions of the net effects of the time that the tissues are in contact, their contact area (A), the temperatures (TBe and TBp) and volume flow rates (Ve and Vp) of blood perfusing the examiner's and patient's skin, epidermal thickness (xe and xp) and thermal conductivity (ke and kp) of both, dermal temperature (TDe and TDp) of both, as well of the net heat exchange rate (QH) between the two tissues. QH is strongly affected by the heat transfer properties of material trapped between the two skin surfaces, for example, air, water, oil, grease, hand lotion, dirt, tissue debris, fabric. [Adams, Steinmetz, Heisey, Holmes and Greenman]

sometimes the dorsal surface of the hands for this assessment. Is one more accurate than the other?

Exercise 7. See whether you can actually 'pick up' any temperature variations, and if so, how your results compare with a, b or c (above) when you palpate for these variations *a quarter of an inch above the body surface.*
(Frymann states: 'Even passing the hand a quarter of an inch above the skin provides information on the surface temperature. An acute lesion area will be unusually warm, an area of long standing, chronic lesion may be unusually cold as compared with the skin in other areas.')

Exercise 8a. Cover the same skin areas, this time assessing for variations in skin friction by lightly running your finger tips across the skin surface (no lubricant). Feel for 'drag', resistance, and so on. If possible also introduce the same variables in which both you and the subject exercise as you repeat the assessment. Note your results, especially if skin friction and temperature variation are noted in the same skin region.

Make a note on a chart of the findings, especially any which indicate both local skin drag/friction characteristics and greater warmth than surrounding tissue.

We need to ask whether an area of skin which 'feels' colder than surrounding skin is really colder (or warmer) or whether in fact this does not relate to higher thermal conductivity coefficient which could be due to an increase in epidermal hydration, as a result of local increase in activity of atrichial sweat glands. This in turn could be due to reflex activity, emotional distress or some local phenomenon.

If the same skin area which palpates as having a different temperature from its surrounding tissue also displays increased skin friction characteristics, the likelihood of increased atrichial sweat gland activity would be strong. We also need to keep in mind our own state of physical and sympathetic activity as it relates to peripheral circulation and epidermal hydration when we palpate:

- Are my hands sweating?
- Have they been sweating?
- Am I relaxed, or anxious?

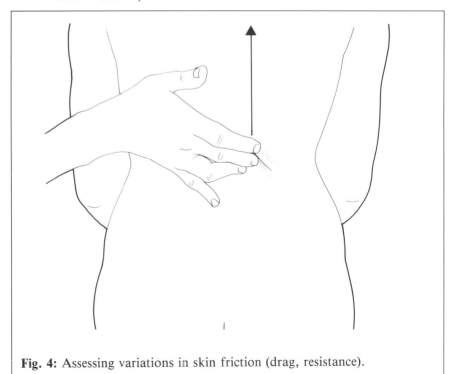

Fig. 4: Assessing variations in skin friction (drag, resistance).

If any of these was affirmative, my thermoreceptors would give potentially inaccurate information as I palpate for temperature variables, a fact which would be compounded were the patient sweating, or the relative ambient humidity or temperature high.

I could also become confused in any attempt I might make to assess tissue texture changes (friction or 'skin drag') were I not aware of the possibility that similar interacting influences (hydration, humidity and so on) can alter 'skin drag' characteristics.

Exercise 8b. If you are even slightly confused as to what you are feeling in this last exercise take off your watch and palpate for skin drag over the skin adjacent to the skin under the strap, and then over that skin. Run your palpating finger(s) from 'dry' skin to 'moist' skin; feel the difference in drag, friction, resistance. Now wait a while – 20 minutes should do – and, without having replaced the watchstrap, perform the exercise again. See how the drag on the skin which was under the strap is now absent; that skin is now the same as the surrounding skin. On another occasion study perceived temperature differences in the skin under a watchstrap, immediately after it is removed, and 20 minutes later, as compared with surrounding skin.

Lewit and his Diagnostic and Treatment Method Using the Skin

Dr Karel Lewit has compiled a treasure house of information in his book *Manipulative Therapy in Rehabilitation of the Motor System*. His discussion of the importance of skin palpation is worth examining in detail here. He points out that it was late in the nineteenth century that Head first reported on increased sensitivity to pinprick sensations in particular zones involved in reflex activity. Unfortunately such a subjective symptom meant that the practitioner was dependent upon accurate feedback from the patient, for whom it was a slow and not particularly comfortable experience.

Lewit also discusses the technique of 'skin-rolling', in which a fold is lifted and rolled forwards between the fingers. Increased resistance is easily noted by the practitioner, as is the fact that wherever reflex activity is operating these folds of skin will also be 'thicker'. Unfortunately this technique is often painful to the patient and is difficult to perform on areas where skin is tightly placed over underlying tissue.

In the German system of connective tissue massage (CTM) the skin is stretched over the underlying tissue by pressing with the fingertips in a direction away from the operator. This is done bilaterally so that variations in the degree of elasticity can be compared from one side of the body to the other. This produces evidence of reflex activity if there is a reduced degree of stretchability when the two sides are compared. Lifting skin folds away from the body is another CTM diagnostic method.

The disadvantages of these methods lie in their fairly general

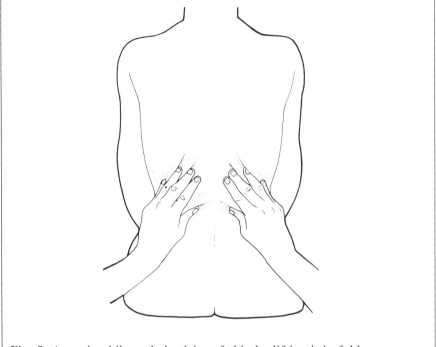

Fig. 5: Assessing bilateral elasticity of skin by lifting it in folds.

indications, although this matters little to those using CTM, since they are usually attempting to identify large reflex zones which relate to organ or system dysfunction, rather than small localised areas of reflex activity.

Lewit reports that he has developed a painless and effective method which is more reliable diagnostically than those mentioned above, and which transforms from diagnostic to therapeutic treatment if the process is prolonged. He calls the method 'skin stretching'. First he stretches the skin with the minimum of force, in order to take up the slack, and takes the stretch to its end-position, where a slight springiness is felt. He does a similar stretch in various directions over the area being assessed. If a hyperalgesic skin zone (HSZ) exists due to reflex input to the area, a 'stiff' resistance is felt after the slack is taken up.

Like has to be compared with like, and it is no use comparing the degree of elasticity available in skin overlaying – say – the lumbar paraspinal muscles with that overlaying the dorsal paraspinal tissues. The first would be relatively 'loose' and the other fairly 'tight' as a natural matter of course. However if one area of dorsal paraspinal skin is compared with another area of dorsal paraspinal skin, and one of these is significantly less elastic than the other, evidence is gained that reflex activity exists below the 'tight' skin.

Treatment of such areas, which initiates a normalizing of the reflex activity which created them, is achieved by maintaining the degree of stretch for a further 10 seconds or so:

If the therapist then holds the stretched skin in end-position, resistance is felt to weaken until normal springing is restored. The hyperalgesic skin zone can then as a rule no longer be detected. *If pain is due to this hyperalgesic skin zone this method is quite as effective as needling, electrostimulation and other similar methods* [My emphasis].

Lewit tells us that this method allows us to diagnose (and treat) even very small reflex areas (HSZ) lying in inaccessible or potentially painful places, such as between the toes, over bony prominences, such as spinous processes, and around scars.

Just what is going on in these HSZs? They sometimes overlay areas affected by viscerosomatic reflex activity or what is known as segmental facilitation, in which the neural structures in any spinal region may respond to repetitive stress factors, of varying types, by becoming hyper-irritable. This produces undesirable consequences locally and in the areas nourished by nerves from that spinal level. We will look at palpation methods for identifying levels of spinal segmental facilitation (other than HSZ) when we examine muscular palpation.

Localized myofascial facilitation also takes place in the development of trigger points, soft tissue hooligans which have the ability to bombard distant tissues with aberrant neural impulses, often of a painful nature, HSZ will be found overlaying active (and also 'embryo' and dormant) trigger points as well as the target zone which the trigger point influences.

Those therapists who are interested in the acupuncture model of treatment will be aware that active points in the meridian system have an area of lowered electrical resistance overlaying them. The location of these would be easily identified by means of Lewit's method of skin stretching (and according to him would respond therapeutically to further stretching, as they would to needling).

There is more detail on the trigger point phenomenon on pp.79–80), including a summary of methods for identifying these common troublemakers, and a reminder of Lewit's methods.

Exercise 9. At first it is necessary to practise this method slowly. Eventually it is possible to move very rapidly over an area which is being searched for evidence of reflex activity (or acupuncture points – the same thing many would say).

Skin Stretching Exercises

Choose two regions which you will search in this way, one an area 3 × 3 in to the side of the dorsal spine, covering the muscular paraspinal region as well as skin over the scapula and/or ribs. The other area should be in the low back/buttock area, much the same size, covering far more elastic, 'loosely fitting', skin. Mark these areas with a skin pencil or felt-tipped pen, and begin the search.

Place your two index fingers adjacent to each other on the skin, side by side or pointing towards each other, with no pressure at all, just a contact touch.

Lightly and slowly separate your fingers, feeling the skin stretch as you do so.

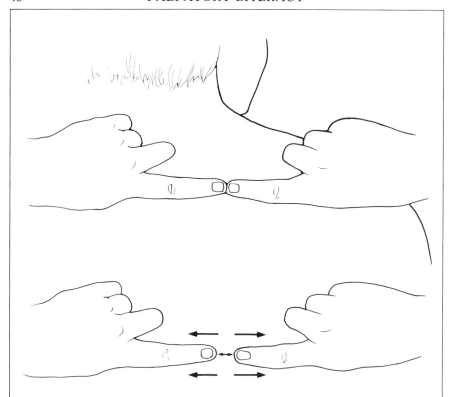

Fig. 6: a) Fingers touch each other directly over skin to be tested – very light skin contact only.
b) Pull apart to assess degree of skin elasticity – compare with neighbouring skin area.

Take the stretch to its 'easy' limit. In other words do not forcibly stretch the skin, just take it to the point where resistance is first noted. This is the 'barrier of resistance' and it should be easily possible with a little more effort to 'spring' the skin further apart to its absolute elastic limit at that time.

Slowly release this and move both fingers $\frac{1}{8}$ in to one side of this first test site, and test again in the same way, *and in the same direction of pull with each finger.*

Perform exactly the same sequence over and over again until the entire 9 square inches of tissue has been searched.

At some points you will sense that the skin is not as elastic as it was on the previous stretch.

This is a hyperalgesic skin zone. Mark it with pencil or pen for future attention.

If you then apply light finger pressure to the centre of that small zone, you will always find a sensitive contracture, which may radiate sensations to a distant site (meaning that it is a trigger point, in which case add to your marking on the skin – or a record card – the direction of the radiating sensation) or may not radiate (meaning that it is either an active acupuncture point, an embryonic trigger point or some other reflex manifestation).

Exercise 10. Now reassess the same skin area but make the direction of each stretch different, perhaps going parallel with the spine rather than vertical to it for example.
See whether you identify the same reflex areas this time.

Exercise 11. Now do a search of the other spinal area which you had marked and note:
    a. The difference in elasticity which is available between skin overlaying the dorsal area and the lumbar/gluteal area.
    b. How it is possible to vary the direction of stretch as you move around the area, and still find yourself able to discriminate between elastic and less elastic skin stretch.
    c. How it is possible to begin to speed up the process so that what took you five minutes of painstakingly careful stretch followed by stretch, can now be achieved in a minute without loss of accuracy.

Exercise 12. Now try to assess the elasticity of skin in difficult areas such as:
    a. The sternum/xyphoid process.
    b. Over the spinous processes.
    c. In the webbing between the toes or fingers.
If you have no available model perform as many of the above exercises as you can on yourself.
Remember that no lubricant should be used during any of these assessments, they are best and most accurately performed 'dry'.
Be careful on hairy areas as this can obviously be uncomfortable.

Exercise 13. Now go back to a marked HSZ, restretch the skin to its barrier, and hold it there for 10 seconds.
Do you feel the skin tightness release?
    Hold it in its new stretched position for a few seconds and then do the same to all other HSZs which you noted in your initial assessments. Now go back and retest the areas and see whether the previously reflexly-restricted skin has regained comparative elasticity.

Exercise 14. Use Lewit's cross-handed ulnar border of the hand contact to assess large skin areas in much the same way, using a firm contact from the little fingers to the wrist. Press lightly down onto the skin with those contacts and separate the hands slightly, seeking to feel for the easy limit of stretch in the skin. Move to an adjacent place and retest, doing this sequentially so that an area such as the back, or thigh is covered. Note any stretches in which there seem to be restriction as compared with neighbouring skin elasticity. This reveals large reflex zones which could relate to organ dysfunction or other neurological evidence. Again practise 'releasing' these restrictions by holding the stretch for 10 seconds or so until a release of tension is felt. Retest to see whether this has indeed made a difference.

Note: The cause of reflex activity which manifests itself as a hyperalgesic skin zone may involve organic, systemic or structural dysfunction, or relate to other longstanding problems. Thus, while skin-stretching release in the manner described may have some input in normalizing function, this is likely to be of only temporary duration unless underlying causes are also dealt with. The methods described above are therefore excellent for identifying reflex activity, but their value in therapeutic terms should be thought of short-term rather than long-term.

Some Further Thoughts on Skin (and Scar Tissue)   In this chapter some very important considerations regarding skin palpation have already been outlined. Some other views on what to look for and expect under different conditions when the skin is palpated are given below.

William Walton (*Journal of the American Osteopathic Association*, August 1971) says:

> In superficial palpation, the operator, using the pads of his fingers, strokes the skin gently, but firmly enough to allow perception, over the area to be examined. There are five types of change to be noted by superficial palpation in both acute and chronic lesions: skin changes, temperature changes, superficial muscle tensions, tenderness and oedema. In acute lesions an actual increase in temperature may be felt in the skin overlaying it, but evidence is vague and extremely fleeting, and not much reliance should be placed on it. The skin overlaying the lesion will feel tense and relatively immobile owing to the congestive effect of the lesion below it. In the chronic lesion, temperature changes may or may not be present... the skin overlaying a chronic lesion may be either normal or reduced as a result of ischaemia of the underlying tissues. This is characteristic of chronic fibrotic change.

Myron Beal D.O. (*Journal of the American Osteopathic Association*, July 1983) has outlined the common paraspinal palpatory findings (mainly involving upper thoracic facilitated segments) relating to patients with acute and chronic cardiovascular disease:

> Skin texture and temperature changes were *not* apparent as consistent, strong findings, compared with the hypertonic state of the deep musculature. In one case of acute myocardial infarction there was an observable increase in the amount of subcutaneous fluid.

John Upledger does not concur with Beal as to skin evidence being unreliable in such diagnosis. He describes use of the skin in localized diagnosis as follows:

> Skin texture changes produced by a facilitated segment are palpable as you lightly drag your fingers over the nearby paravertebral area of the back. I usually do skin drag evaluation moving from the top of the neck to the sacral area in one motion. Where your fingertips drag on the skin (see

discussion of this phenomenon earlier in this chapter) you will probably find a facilitated segment. After several repetitions, with increased force, the affected area will appear redder than nearby areas. This is the 'red reflex'.

Muscles and connective tissues at this level will: 1) have a 'shotty' feel (like BBs under the skin); 2) be more tender to palpation; 3) be tight, and tend to restrict vertebral motion; and 4) exhibit tenderness of the spinous processes when tapped by fingers or a rubber hammer.

(Craniosacral Therapy: Beyond the Dura)

The difference of opinion between Beal and Upledger may have resulted from different palpatory methods, or, more likely, simply because Beal finds the evidence from the muscles more reliable (see Chapter 4). He does after all say that the skin evidence is not 'as consistent' as the muscle evidence, not that skin evidence is not available.

Scars
Karel Lewit M.D. brings into focus yet another skin phenomenon which is often overlooked, the scar (*Manipulation in Rehabilitation of the Motor System*). In his discussion of conditions which are resistant to treatment, or where symptoms don't seem to be explained by findings, he suggests we look for scar tissue:

The German literature uses the term *storungsfeld* – 'focus of disturbance'. This is frequently an old scar after injury or operation, often a tonsillectomy scar. This focus-scar is usually tender on examination, with pain spots and surrounded by a hyperalgesic zone.

Such scars may act as 'saboteurs', he believes, requiring special attention. He suggests deep palpation for pain spots, assessing for increased resistance ('adhesions') as well as for HSZ, by skin stretching. If release of the skin by stretching fails to resolve the situation (simple skin-stretching is usually very successful with scars, says Lewit), needling (into pain spots) or local infiltration injections may be called for. When treatment has been successful the local skin resistance and the pain spots should vanish, and the patient's symptoms should start improving.

Upledger and Vredevoogd (*Craniosacral Therapy*) discuss scar tissue, illustrating its importance with the example of a patient with chronic migraine headaches which resulted from chronic fascial drag produced by an appendectomy scar: 'Deep pressure medially on the scar produced the headache; deep pressure laterally caused relief of the headache. Mobilization of the scar was performed by sustained and deep but gentle pressure.' This resulted in freedom from headaches according to these respected authors, who add: 'Spontaneous relief of low back pain, menstrual disorders and chronic and recurrent cervical somatic dysfunction also occured following cicatrix [scar] mobilization.' The influence of fascia on soft tissue function and dysfunction will be considered in the next chapter.

Exercise 15. Palpate a scar. Feel the tissue itself, and see how the surrounding tissue associates with it. If possible palpate a recent and a very old scar. Compare them. See if local tenderness exists around the scar. See how the skin elasticity varies when this is the case. Can you release the skin by sustained painless stretching?

Connective Tissue Massage Diagnostic Method

In the discussion of Lewit's hyperalgesic skin zones earlier in this chapter, brief mention was made of the German system *bindegewebsmassage* or connective tissue massage. This was named by a physical therapist, Elizabeth Dicke, in her book *Meine Bindegewebsmassage*, published in Stuttgart in 1954. The methods used – the application of patterns of repetitive dry-contact, strong friction stroke, aimed at evoking reflex responses, do not concern us in this study. However, the diagnostic methods used to identify areas (zones) suitable for treatment are significant.

Dicke's method of diagnosis is discussed by Irmgard Bischof and Ginette Elmiger in their chapter 'Connective Tissue Massage' in Sidney Licht's book *Massage, Manipulation and Traction*:

a. Both hands, applied flat, displace the subcutaneous tissues simultaneously against the fascia, with small to and fro pushes. The degree of displacement possible will depend upon tension of the tissues. It is important that symmetrical areas [i.e. both sides of body] be examined simultaneously.
b. By pulling away a skin fold from the fascia, the degree of tissue tension

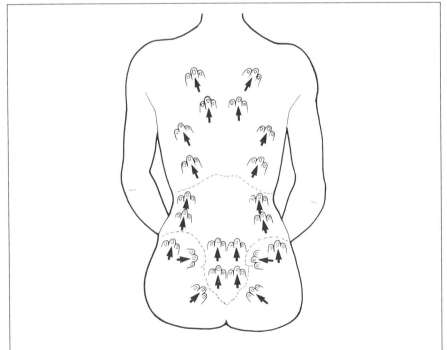

Fig. 7: Testing tissue mobility by bilaterally 'pushing' skin with fingertip.

and displacement may be determined. Three different levels of displacement are distinguished:

1) the most superficial displacement occurs between skin and subcutaneous tissues and is easier to find in children and in old people because the displacement is slight;

2) the main displacement occurs between the subcutaneous tissue and the fascia;

3) the deepest displacement layer is between the fascia and the interstitial connective tissue. The movement is most evident upon large, flat areas such as the lumbosacral area, on the sacrum, and in regions of the tensor fascia lata.

Apart from this diagnostic method the system uses a further 'diagnostic stroke' which employs a two-finger contact (patient seated, as a rule) which runs longitudinally, paravertebrally, starting at the level of L5 up to the level of the 7th cervical spinous process. As the stroke (pull) starts, the upper layers of displacement are superficial and gentle; they are followed by a slower deeper stroke which pulls on subcutaneous tissue and fascia. Displacement of the deeper tissue, as well as interstitial tissue, is accomplished by a deep and slow pull along the same 'track'.

This highlights an important point, namely that the desired depth effect is obtained by the *speed* of the strokes *as well as the amount of pressure*. This is true also of neuromuscular technique, and is a most useful tip for those attempting to enhance palpatory skills. Slow down, the information is there and it cannot be hurried. What should the stroke show?

Healthy tissue elevates or 'mounds' ahead of the stroking digits (2 to 3 centimetres ahead). When an area of resistance is reached, increased tension is felt and further displacement of the skin becomes difficult or impossible. Folds of skin will be formed in front of the advancing stroke in such areas and the mass will become larger. The progress of the stroke will also become slower, as compared with the stroke across healthy tissue. Factors such as age of patient, constitutional state, posture and the area being tested, will all alter the anticipated findings.

It is easier to displace skin against underlying tissue in slim individuals, with little fatty tissue. Obese individuals have a higher fat and water content subcutaneously, making displacement more difficult.

Dicke pointed out that even before use of the diagnostic stroke it is often possible to see reflex areas. They are characterized by being retracted or elevated. Retracted bands of tissue are commonly seen in areas such as the neck, lower thoracic border and over the pelvic and gluteal areas. Depressed or flattened areas are seen over the thorax, the scapulae and between the thoracic spine and the scapula as well as over the upper iliac tissues and the sacrum. Flat elevations are visible in many cases around the 7th cervical spinous process, on the outer border of the scapulae or around the sacrum.

These raised or depressed tissue areas are not amenable to dissipation by massage and represent chronic reflex activity. They are considered to be viscero-cutaneous reflexes (viscero-somatic in other words) resulting from altered blood supply leading to colloidal changes in the cells and tissues.

What is revealed by these diagnostic strokes is alteration in vascular skin reaction, tissue tension, tissue density, tissue sensitivity and often tissue displacement; the relevance of these changes is hopefully clearer now that the subject of tissue hydration has been covered. Valuable clinical evidence can be gathered using these strokes and 'pushes'. For a deeper understanding of this system Dicke's work should be studied in depth. Fortunately this system is now taught world-wide by her followers and is much used by physical therapists, massage therapists and some doctors, osteopaths and chiropractors who employ soft tissue methods. We now have something of an answer (only the beginning though, as will become clear) to questions such as those of osteopathic physician Paul Van Allen D.O. (Academy of Applied Osteopathy Yearbook 1963), who asks:

> How does one palpate? This seems too absurdly simple to bother with an answer. Yet Pottenger wrote half a book on *Light Touch Palpation in Visceral Disease*, without pretending to be exhaustive. 'Stroking' is a means of determining skin texture, a means of setting up vibrations in the tissues. Pottenger was able by this means to outline the heart, liver, spleen or an area of consolidation in the lung.

Refer to Exercise 5 in Chapter 2 for a method for enhancement of specific palpatory skills relating to assessment of 'density' of tissues, suggested by Dr Van Allen. See how long it takes you to palpate the borders of an organ using light touch.

Exercise 16. Putting it all together: if you carefully noted your findings when performing the tests for temperature variation and 'skin drag' you should now be able to compare those notes with your findings using Lewit's method of identification of hyperalgesic skin zones using skin stretching. Also compare these findings with those using Dicke's method.

Obviously such comparisons will only be valid if you have used the same subject/model. If not, on a subsequent occasion do ensure that you use all the skin assessment variations described on the same subject, and compare results as you use the following: direct palpation for heat variations; assessment of heat variables a quarter of an inch above the surface; light stroking for 'skin drag' variations; skin stretching for identification of HSZ; connective tissue 'diagnostic stroke' method.

Do these findings agree? They should. If not try again, and again. Incorporate as many of these methods as you can into your pattern of assessment.

Is it a Muscle or a Joint Problem?

- Is this patient's pain a soft tissue or a joint problem?
- How can we very rapidly make this differentiation?

There are several simple screening tests we can apply, in answer to these questions, based on the work of Professor Freddy Kaltenborn, of Norway (*Mobilization of the Extremity Joints*).

1. Does passive stretching (traction) of the painful area increase the level of pain?
If so it is probably of soft tissue origin (extra-articular).

2. Does compression of the painful area increase the pain?
If so it is probably of joint origin (intra-articular) involving tissues belonging to that anatomical joint.

3. If active (controlled by the patient) movement in one direction produces pain (and/or is restricted), while passive (controlled by the operator) movement in the *opposite* direction, also produces pain (and/or is restricted), the contractile tissues (muscle, ligament etc) are implicated.
This can be confirmed by resisted tests, described below.

4. If active movement and passive movement in the *same* direction produce pain (and/or restriction), joint dysfunction is probable.
This can be confirmed by use of traction and compression (and gliding) tests of the joint (see notes on Joint play, p.151).

Resisted tests are used to assess both strength and painful responses to muscle contraction, either from the muscle or its tendinous attachment. This involves producing a maximal contraction of the suspected muscle while the joint is kept immobile somewhere near the middle of range position. No joint motion should be allowed to occur. This is done after Test 3 above to confirm a soft tissue dysfunction rather than a joint involvement. Before doing the resisted test it is wise to perform the compression test to clear any suspicion of joint involvement.

If, on resisted testing (according to Professor J. Cyriax, *Textbook of Orthopaedic Medicine*), the muscle seems strong and also painful there is no more than a minor lesion/dysfunction of the muscle or its tendon.

If it is weak and painful, there is a more serious lesion/dysfunction of the muscle or tendon.

If it is weak and painless, there may be a neurological lesion, or the tendon has ruptured.

A normal muscle tests strong and pain-free. Test all these statements on conditions of known origin.

Obviously in many instances soft tissue dysfunction will accompany (precede or follow on from) joint dysfunction. Joint involvement is less likely in the early stages of soft tissue dysfunction, than (for example) in the chronic stages of muscle shortening. There are few joint conditions, acute or chronic, without some soft tissue involvement. The tests described above will give a strong indication though, as to whether the major involvement in such a situation is of soft or osseous structures.

Examples of a joint assessment involving compression, would be the ones described by Blower and Griffin (*Annals of Rheumatic Disease*, 1984, 43: 192–5) for sacroiliac dysfunction. This showed that pressure applied over the lower half of the sacrum, or over the anterior superior iliac spines, were diagnostic of sacroiliac problems (possibly ankylosing spondylitis) if pain was produced in the sacrum and buttocks. Soft tissue dysfunction would not produce painful responses with this type of compression test.

Note: Lumbar pain is not significant if it occurs on sacral pressure, as this action causes movement of the lumbosacral joint, and to some extent throughout the whole lumbar spine.

Chapter 4

Palpating for Changes in Muscle Structure

Unlike the skin, which is there for us to see as well as touch, once we begin to explore the inner regions of the body and try to deduce just what state the soft tissues are in, far greater skills are required if we are successfully to gather information as to the current tissue state, the likely causes and probable prognosis.

General guidance can be given as to what superficial muscular tissues *should* feel like under given conditions, and it is not difficult to learn to read such information by gentle palpation. But it is not just the relative state of tone, tension, contraction, flaccidity and so on which need to be assessed, important though these factors are; there are also fluid fluctuations through connective tissue, and other rhythmic patterns, which indicate the degree of normality or otherwise of the soft tissues, as well as having wider implications. In order to make sense of these fluid movements when it comes to palpating at greater depth – or understanding more subtle energy – we need to employ fairly refined skills.

Some of these have been well explored and explained by diligent researchers, among them John Upledger D.O. who discusses the mechanics which govern the vital physiological motions in some of the exercises in Chapter 2; Rollin Becker D.O. in his articles on 'Diagnostic Touch' in the 1963, 1964 and 1965 *Yearbooks of the Academy of Applied Osteopathy*; Fritz Smith M.D. in his book *Inner Bridges: A Guide to Energy Movement and Body Structure*; and Stanley Lief D.C. D.O., the prime developer of neuromuscular technique, whose work has been described in my book, *Soft Tissue Manipulation*.

The techniques and exercises based on the work of these and other developers of the art and science of palpation have expanded the potential for skilful assessment of the pathophysiological state of the muscles and other soft tissues. In this chapter we will be reviewing methods aimed at determining *structural* changes in the soft tissues (increased tone, shortening, fibrous development, periosteal pain points, trigger points and so on) whereas in the next chapter it is the palpation of *functional* changes – those which can be 'read' through muscles and other soft tissues – which will be considered.

Why Changes Occur in the Soft Tissues

Before we delve into methods of palpation of soft tissue structures, we should briefly review the reasons why the changes we are trying to evaluate occur. A host of interacting factors have the ability to increase muscular tone, including stress response, postural anomalies and overload, repetitive physical actions (sport, occupation hobbies and so on), emotional distress, trauma, structural factors (congenital short leg, cranial distortion at birth) visceral and other reflex activity. These can be summarized as *overuse*, *misuse*, and *abuse* of the musculoskeletal structures.

When tone in a muscle is initially increased for any length of time a degree of local irritation results, due to two factors:

1. Local tissue hypoxia or ischaemia, in which states inadequate oxygenation of the tissues occurs due to the increase in tone.
2. Relative inadequacy of drainage and removal of metabolic waste products, for the same reason.

This combination leads first to fatigue, then to irritation, and in some instances to inflammation over time. This might be termed the 'acute' phase of the body-response to any persistent increase in tone. During this stage pain would often be a feature, which in turn would create a cycle of even greater tone and therefore more pain. Palpation would show the tissues to be warmer than surrounding tissue, possibly oedematous, and usually very sensitive or painful.

This phase may be equated with the alarm stage in Selye's general adaptation syndrome (GAS). Indeed all elements of the GAS can be scaled down to a local level (a single muscle, or joint, for example) in which the same stages are passed through (alarm, adaptation, collapse). This is then referred to as the local adaptation syndrome (LAS).

As would be expected according to both GAS and LAS, after the acute phase would come the phase of adaptation. In the muscular sense this means that if increased tone is held for longer than a few weeks a chronic stage evolves. This is characterized by a beginning of structural change in the supporting tissues with the development of fibrotic alterations. Some see these as an 'organizing' response, in which tone is replaced by concrete supportive bands. The body is adapting to the seemingly permanent demand for increased tone in the musculature.

The degree of relative ischaemia hypoxia and toxic debris retention increases at this stage, varying from person to person (and region to region) in relation to features such as age, amount of exercise, nutritional status and so on. Any pain noted would probably have a more deep, aching quality. Palpation would reveal a more fibrous, stringy texture and other palpable changes; it is during this adaptation stage that early signs would be noted of trigger point development, in which discrete areas of the affected soft tissues would evolve into localized areas of facilitation.

Highly sensitive, discrete and palpable tissue changes would be found which are themselves capable of sending noxious impulses to a distant target area where pain and a new crop of trigger points would develop.

Bands of stress fibres would become evident in the hypertonic tissues and the muscles affected in this way would begin to place increasing degrees of tension on their tendons and osseous insertions. (See notes on connective tissue diagnostic methods in Chapter 3 for commentary on palpable bands and zones).

As this occurs tendon changes begin and the same pattern of the acute phase, followed by the adaptation phase and progressing on to degenerative changes is observed. As these stresses begin to affect the tendons and as these begin to adapt it is usually possible to palpate very tender periosteal pain points, or to note early signs of joint dysfunction. The natural sequence described by Selye from acute phase to the adaptation phase (which can last many years) and ultimately when adaptive capabilities are exhausted, the final phase of degeneration and disease, will be the natural consequence of any unrelieved chronic hypertonicity. This could take the form of arthritic joint changes or chronic muscular or other soft tissue dysfunction.

As will become clear the abbreviated pattern of LAS, outlined above, has quite different effects in postural muscles than in more active phasic muscles. Postural muscles (see p.95 for a fuller explanation of this concept) when chronically abused, misused, overused, will tend to shorten and eventually to contract. Phasic muscles, however, when faced with the same insults, will tend to weaken not shorten.

The task of the palpating hand(s) is to uncover the locality, nature, degree and if possible the age, of the soft tissue changes which take place in the sequence outlined above. As we palpate we need to ask:

- Is this palpable change acute or chronic (or – as is often the case – an acute phase of a chronic condition)?
- How do these palpable soft tissue changes relate to the patient's symptom pattern?
- Are these palpable changes part of a pattern of stress-induced change which can be mapped?
- Are these soft tissue changes painful, and if so what is the nature of that pain?
- Are these palpable changes active reflexly, are they trigger points (do they refer symptoms elsewhere)?
- Are they the result of trigger points elsewhere, or of other reflex
- activity (see viscero-somatic reflex activity p.61)?
- Are these changes present in a postural or phasic muscle group? (See p.95 for methods of assessing shortened postural muscles.)
- Are these palpable changes the result of joint restriction ('blockage', subluxation, lesion) or are they contributing to such dysfunction?
- In other words we need to ask ourselves *What am I feeling, and what does it mean?*

Viola Frymann helps to illuminate the need for some thought as to how deeper palpation might be carried out as we search for such changes, acute or chronic:

> A slightly firmer approach brings the examiner into communication with the superficial muscles to determine their tone, their turgor, their metabolic state. Penetrating more deeply, similar study of the deeper muscle layers is possible (and) the state of the fascial sheaths and condensations may be noted.

The words 'firmer' and 'penetrating more deeply', if taken too literally could lead to 'counter-productive' palpation; if these recommendations were to involve a noticeable increase in applied pressure, two negative possibilities might eventuate. First there could be a defensive retraction of the palpated tissues, tensing superficial musculature, making assessment difficult or its interpretation invalid; and secondly there is likely to be a lessening of sensitivity as pressure increases on the surface of the palpating digit, especially if it is sustained for more than a short time, greatly affecting the accuracy of perception.

Different solutions have been found in order to overcome these problems. In Lief's system of neuromuscular evaluation, which will be outlined later in this chapter, these problems are largely overcome by use of what is termed 'variable' pressure, in which the digital contact matches the resistance it meets from the tissues. A subtle and effective method is therefore available for fairly deep assessment of soft tissues status, with little evidence of protective tensing by the tissues, or of much loss of sensitivity in the thumb or finger contact.

Others have approached this problem differently, most notably John Upledger with his 'melding' and synchronization approach, which leads to the palpating instrument doing 'exactly what the patient's body is doing and would otherwise be doing, even if you weren't there'.

Rollin Becker D.O. uses what he describes as a 'fulcrum' palpation technique, which increases perception of tissues at depth without greatly increasing pressure on the skin surface. Fritz Smith M.D. makes his assessments in yet another way, using among other methods, what he terms a 'half-moon' vector contact. The first section of this chapter will look at palpation of structure (as opposed to the palpation of function involved in assessment of rhythmic fluctuations and pulses) including various ideas and recommendations for palpation of the soft tissues, derived from a number of prominent physicians and researchers from various schools and disciplines, including Magoun, Tilley, Lief, Nimmo, Dicke, Lewit and Beal. This will be followed by a summary of recommended methods for sequential assessment of shortened postural muscles, the importance of which will be explained as we progress.

Interspersed amongst this review material will be a number of exercises which can enhance sensitivity when practising one or other of these methods. There is inevitably going to be a degree of overlap in the concepts of these innovators of palpatory (and therapeutic) technique, but each has a unique insight into the needs of the practitioner who is trying to make sense of physical problems as they 'read' the body.

It is suggested that all the methods outlined in this and the next chapter be attempted, practised, and assessed for their individual degree of usefulness. Many therapists use all these methods (and others) in appropriate settings.

Jiri and Vaclav Dvorak outline their basic requirements for sound palpation of structures of the musculoskeletal system in their book *Manual Medicine: Diagnostics*. They insist that a healthy anatomical structure cannot be differentiated from surrounding structures whereas 'a pathologically altered structure however, can be exactly differentiated from the surrounding healthy tissue'.

Palpation and Assessment of Structure

Apart from starting to palpate from the site where the patient localizes the symptom (usually pain), their other major emphasis is on the therapist having a 'three dimensional anatomical perception' of what is being palpated, a useful description to emphasize the need for a sound anatomical knowledge. Such knowledge leads, they suggest, to the application of 'adequate pressure with regard to area, force and direction' as 'the muscles, ligaments and other structures are located above and next to each other in the specific topographical region'.

They suggest beginning at the site of pain, localizing this and palpating precisely for hard, bony structures; along tendons for information about the insertion; comparing not with symmetrically placed sites but with 'locations with the same anatomical arrangement and sites undergoing no changes'; differentiating from similar changes in adjacent structures by palpating the course, shape and opposite poles of attachment (origin and insertion) of such structures; identification of myotendinosis by use of stroking and pressing palpation, performed perpendicular to the direction of the fibres until origins and insertions are reached.

Compare this description with the diagnostic methods of Lief's neuromuscular technique, and Nimmo's methods, as outlined below, and decide which approach best suits your way of working.

The Facilitated Segment

Harold Magoun is renowned as one of the giants of osteopathic medicine, both clinically and theoretically. Writing in the *Journal of the American Osteopathic Association* (December 1948, 'Osteopathic Diagnosis and Therapy for the General Practitioner') Magoun made an important contribution to our understanding of the structural analysis of muscular tissues. Describing what the seeking practitioner will uncover, he says:

> What should palpation reveal? First he finds that the soft tissues are abnormal. Then he must determine if the condition is a primary lesion (local) or a viscerosomatic reflex. While these are often combined, especially if not recent, the differential diagnosis is most important.

He makes the distinction between what will be palpated if the cause of altered soft tissue feel is a local problem or if it is of reflex origin. The primary lesion involves mainly the deep muscles, producing an *inert and irregular* rigor, if of long standing the superficial tissues may be atonic or stringy. The hypersensitivity is usually limited to the deeper tissues. Magoun points out that there may be oedema in the connective tissue and that if the condition is years old 'fibrous degeneration takes place with overgrowth, of connective tissue, calcification, thickening of the periosteum and so on'.

He then differentiates the above description from what would obtain if the cause of tissue change were of reflex (organ disease) origin:

> The uncomplicated viscerosomatic reflex is manifested by a concentration of both superficial and deep tissues, both of which are hypersensitive to the same degree [only deep tissues are expected to be sensitive in primary lesion condition]. *This continuous contraction or exaggerated tone makes the tissues hard and tense in a regular homogenous manner* (My emphasis).

Compare this description with that of the research findings of Beal, some 35 years later, when he makes clear the difference in general somatic effect of such a reflex change:

> There is no change in the nutrition such as brings about a wasting or ropy condition of the muscles; there is no change in the circulation so as to produce haemorrhage or oedema; there is no ligamentous thickening or fibrositis or oedema about the joint.

He rightly directs attention to correction of viscerosomatic reflex activity by dealing with the causes of the dysfunction of the affected organ, which might involve nutritional, manipulative or surgical intervention.

> **Exercise 1.** If it is possible to examine a patient with known visceral disease (cardiovascular, digestive) palpate the superficial and deeper musculature paraspinally, to see whether a local segment can be identified which matches the description given by Magoun. There should be superficial and deep contraction of tissues on one or both sides of the spine, at an appropriate segmental level (see p.63 for Tilley's suggested sites), both layers being hypersensitive. If possible compare findings with those paraspinally adjacent to a known structural problem where only the deeper tissues should be contracted and sensitive.

Tilley and Korr on the Facilitated Segment

R. McFarlane Tilley D.O. summarized his ideas on digital palpation of the spine as follows (*1961 Academy of Applied Osteopathy Yearbook*).

> 1. Light palpation to discover areas of increased moisture on the skin surface, indicating increased sweat gland activity.
> 2. Moderate friction of the skin by heavier stroking to elicit 'red reaction'.
> 3. Deep palpation to elicit muscular tension and tenderness of tissues upon pressure.

He follows this with an examination of range of motion and restrictions. Stress patterns may develop for any number of physical or emotional reasons, he states, as a result of which spinal nerve pathways and cord centres become facilitated (hyper-reactive). When this occurs related spinal musculature become palpably stressed; reflex relationships may be involved, including both vicerosomatic and somaticovisceral pathways. Professor Irvin Korr (*1976 Academy of Applied Osteopathy Yearbook*) has compared any facilitated area of the spine to a 'neurological lens', in which stress factors which impinge upon any aspect of the body or mind are automatically targeted through the facilitated segment, further focusing and intensifying activity through its neurological structures.

A simple diagnostic palpation method for 'compressing' or 'springing' the paraspinal tissues will be discussed below, by means of which the likelihood of a facilitated segment being present can usually be readily confirmed. The common palpatory feature of segmental facilitation as it manifests in the paraspinal musculature is of relative rigidity and tenderness, as compared with the segments above and below. As a rule this will involve two or more adjacent segments, rather than just one local segment. If this rigidity results from visceral pathology it will fail to respond – other than for a very short time – to any physical treatment applied to the muscles or joints involved. These rigid muscular states can however be a useful prognostic indicator of change, for better or worse, as therapy is applied to the dysfunctioning organ in question.

Tilley lists the *possible* meanings of such facilitation in various spinal regions, based on osteopathic clinical observations:

- Myocardial ischaemia: rigid musculature in any two adjacent segments between T1 and T4 (usually left, but not essentially so).
- Cardiopulmonary pathology: any two adjacent segments of muscular paraspinal rigidity in the upper thoracic spine, either side or bilaterally.
- Duodenal pathology: any two adjacent segments of muscular paraspinal rigidity and tenderness, right side thoracic spine, levels 6, 7 and 8.
- Pancreatic dysfunction: any two adjacent segments of muscular paraspinal rigidity and tenderness, bilaterally, thoracics 6, 7, 8 and 9.
- Liver and gall bladder: any two adjacent segments of muscular paraspinal rigidity and tenderness, right side thoracics 8, 9 and 10.
- Chronic fatigue related to 'Adrenal exhaustion' or stress: any two adjacent segments of muscular paraspinal rigidity and tenderness in thoracics 9, 10, 11 and 12.
- Renal disease: tenderness and painful on pressure, aggravated by percussion, thoracics 11, 12 and lumbars 1, 2.
- Female and male reproductive organ problems: lumbosacral area tenderness or rigidity.

Note: It is important to differentiate between segmental facilitation and spinal 'splinting' which occurs as a result of underlying pathology such as TB spine, vertebral metastasis (primary or secondary) and osteoporosis. Splinting such as this will usually be more widespread than the two adjacent segments associated with segmental facilitation. No attempt should be made to reduce such splinting, which is protective.

Exercise 2. On a suitable patient/model follow Tilley's recommendation to lightly palpate for signs of increased moisture (sweat gland activity) and 'drag', followed by heavier stroking to elicit the 'red response'. Where this is observed palpate more deeply for deep muscular tension and tenderness.

Beal's Method for Identifying Segmental Facilitation by Palpation
Myron Beal D.O., Professor in the Department of Family Medicine at Michigan State University College of Osteopathic Medicine conducted a study in which over a hundred patients with diagnosed cardiovascular disease were examined for patterns of spinal segment involvement.

Around 90 per cent had 'segmental dysfunction in two or more adjacent vertebrae from T1 to T5, on the left side'. More than half also had left side C2 dysfunction. Beal reports that the estimation of the intensity of the spinal dysfunction correlated strongly with the degree of pathology noted (ranging from myocardial infarction, ischaemic heart disease and hypertensive cardiovascular disease, to coronary artery disease).

He further reports that the greatest intensity of the cardiac reflex occurred at T2 and T3 on the left. The texture of the soft tissues, as described by Beal ('Palpatory testing for somatic dysfunction in patients with cardiovascular disease', *Journal of American Osteopathic Association*, July 1983), is of interest: Skin and temperature changes were not apparent as consistent strong findings compared with the hypertonic state of the deep musculature.' The major palpatory finding for muscle was of hypertonicity of the superficial and deep paraspinal muscles with fibrotic thickening. Tenderness was usually obvious, although this was not specifically assessed in this study. Superficial hypertonicity lessened when the patient was supine making assessment of deeper tissue states easier in that position.

Palpation Method for Identifying Thoracic Areas of Segmental Facilitation
With the patient supine, the thoracic spine is examined by the operator sliding the fingers under the transverse processes, and applying an anterior compressive force, assessing the status of the superficial and deep paraspinal tissues and the response of the transverse process to an anterior, compressive, springing force (hence Beal's term of 'compression test' for this method). This compression is performed one segment at a time progressing down the spine, until control becomes difficult. It is also possible to perform the test with patient seated or side-lying, though neither are as effective as the supine position.

Exercise 3. As an exercise in developing this particular skill it is suggested that some time be spent carefully springing the thoracic paraspinal tissues (and transverse processes) with a supine model/patient/partner. If possible try to perform such palpation on people with and without known cardiovascular (or other visceral) dysfunction in order to develop a degree of discrimination between normal and abnormal tissue states of this sort.

Exercise 4. Use all the elements in Exercises 1, 2 and 3 of this chapter on the same patient at the same time, and see which methods produce the most reliable evidence of viscerosomatic reflex activity.

When considering paraspinal soft tissues we must not forget the very small intersegmental muscles in this area which would be dramatically affected by such facilitation. Korr reminds us:

> Intersegmental mobility is very finely tuned by the small and easily forgotten muscles that run from segment to segment. Their critical role is not always appreciated in considerations of longstanding degenerative changes. We can see that the large muscles, for example the erector spinae group, initiate large movements, but which mediates the translation of forces from one segment to the next? What concentrates the force of a particular motion at one particular locality, not once but a hundred thousands times in 20 years or so?
>
> The intersegmental muscles are the conditioning agents and if their function is disturbed the result may be a change in the tracking characteristics at that particular junction, which in time will show impaired function.

Korr also reminds us that the more active a muscle is in fine movement, the greater the number of muscle spindles there will be present (as in the hands). He goes on:

> Studies such as those involving the deep occipital muscles have indicated roughly the same ratio between spindles in the small and large muscles [as in the hand i.e. 26:1.5]. *Although disturbances here are not apparent on routine examination they are detectable when the clinician has a well-developed palpatory sense.* Locating these disorders and modifying or removing them, insofar as possible, is a most logical and important element in preventive medicine (My emphasis).

It may be useful to consider how the physicians in Beal's study (p.64) described what they actually felt. In a separate study of palpatory reliability by Hugo Rosero *et al.*, *Journal of the American Osteopathic Association*, February 1987, the terms most commonly used by palpating physicians to describe their findings in this type of condition were examined. Sixteen descriptive terms were provided for their use. Only five were consistently used to indicate what they were feeling on palpation: resistant (firm, tense); temperature warm; ropiness (cord-like); heavy musculature (increased density) and oedematous. Of these 'resistant' and 'temperature warm' were most commonly used.

Did you feel the 'resistant and warm' tissues when doing exercises 1, 2, 3 and 4? If not try again.

Supportive Chinese Evidence

Paraspinally, in Traditional Chinese Medicine, lie the Bladder Meridian points. In a study of 33 patients with gastro or duodenal ulceration some significant findings were produced. These patients were scheduled for subtotal gastrectomy (Yuan Cunxin *et al. Journal of Traditional Chinese Medicine 6*(4) 1986), but before operation they were palpated paraspinally:

> The patients lay on their sides and were palpated 2 or 3 times with the physician's thumb along the medial line of the Urinary Bladder Channel of Foot Taiyang ($1\frac{1}{2}$ of the subject's thumbwidths lateral to, and parallel with, spinous processes) from above downward. The location of any tender spots (hereafter referred to as reaction spots) and the shape and location of any palpable mass under the reaction point were recorded.

The researchers recorded the degree of pressure required to elicit tenderness on these points and also applied pressure 10 cm lateral to the reaction points as a means of establishing a control for comparison. A week after surgery the same reaction points (and the control points) were reassessed.

Before surgery 89.4 per cent of the patients with peptic ulcer had reaction points overlaying traditional acupuncture points Pishu (U.B.20) and Weishu (U.B.21) at spinal levels T9–T12. The palpated findings at that time are described as 'mainly cord-like in shape, soft and mobile', averaging 1.19 sq.cm. in size. At the reassessment these were scarcely palpable and required far greater pressure to elicit tenderness (from a mean of 1.89 kilograms of pressure to a mean of 3.22 kilograms of pressure. The pressure required to 'hurt' the control points hardly varied pre- and post-operatively, around $3\frac{1}{2}$ kilograms).

The significance of these findings is as follows:

> a. Somatic reference points resulting from visceral pathology are palpable.
> b. The findings may range from rigidity, if segmental facilitation is operating, to 'soft and cord-like' if it is not.
> c. Both the sensitivity and the structural changes alter or vanish in tandem with changes or disappearance of the visceral disease.

Such palpatory findings therefore have prognostic value.

The Chinese study also examined the effect of needling similar reactive points relating to stomach pain unrelated to ulceration, in over 100 patients. They achieved a 93.8 per cent response rate (improvement or 'cure') which led them to claim:

> Anomalies of internal viscera are manifested on the body surface, and needling these surface reaction points (acupuncture points) produces regulating effects on visceral functions and so can correct the anomaly.

Whether this claim can be substantiated or not is debatable, since causes [smoking, stress, diet and so on] are unlikely to be corrected by acupuncture alone. However a beneficial influence can certainly be claimed for the methods described.

Palpating skills can therefore provide evidence, from the paraspinal muscles, of visceral dysfunction, and we have Beal's 'compression' test as a guide to what to anticipate if pathology is marked and involves the spinal segment itself.

Lief's Neuromuscular Technique
Neuromuscular technique (NMT) evolved in Europe in the 1930s as a blend of traditional Ayurvedic (Indian) techniques and methods derived from other sources. The therapist who created this method of combined diagnostic and therapeutic value was Stanley Lief D.O., D.C. He and his son Peter (also a D.C. graduate of National College of Chiropractic, Chicago) and his cousin Boris Chaitow D.C. (also from National) developed the techniques now known as NMT into an excellent and economical diagnostic (and therapeutic) tool. Our attention will be focused on the palpatory diagnostic potential of NMT, for here is a system which allows methodical, sequential, systematic, controlled combing of the major accessible (to palpating digits) sites of trigger points and other forms of localized soft tissue dysfunction.

Other methods commonly used in seeking out trigger points, such as those advocated by Raymond Nimmo D.C. (taught in the United States, confusingly enough, as 'neuromuscular technique') do not have this feature of systematic, sequential, *comprehensive* pattern of search which leaves little to chance. If there are trigger points present, NMT ('European' version) will find them.

Within shortened muscles (see p.95 for a sequence of assessment for short muscles) and within weakened ones as well, there are often to be found an abundant crop of palpable, localized, discrete, sensitive areas of altered structure, which may or may not be active trigger points, but which are all potential trigger points.

All palpable, sensitive, tissue changes are of importance in palpatory analysis. Some will be trigger points but even if such 'points' are not referring symptoms elsewhere they are of potential diagnostic value. (They could be points described in some other system, such as Chapman's neurolymphatic reflexes or Bennet's neurovascular reflexes, or active acupuncture points, or Jones's 'tender' points). All of these would also be characterized by overlying skin being less elastic than surrounding tissue (see Chapter 3) or by having a measurable degree of lowered electrical resistance.

One simple definition of a trigger point is that it is a *palpable*, sensitive, localized structure, within the soft tissues, which is sending *aberrant*, *noxious*, *neurological* impulses to a distant site and which, on pressure, refers symptoms – usually involving pain, but with other symptoms possible – to this predictable target area.

Doctors Janet Travell and David Simons, authors of the finest exposition on myofascial trigger points to date, *The Trigger Point Manual* give a broader definition which is summarized on p.79.)

The major sites of these self-perpetuating trouble-makers (trigger points) are often close to the origins and insertions of muscles, and this

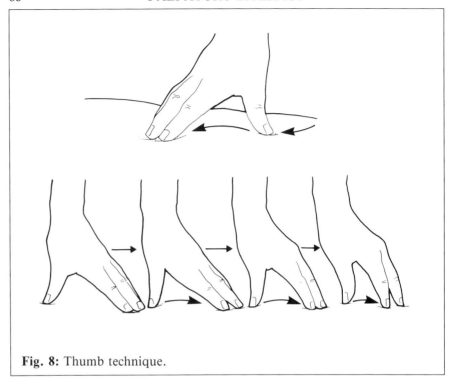

Fig. 8: Thumb technique.

is where NMT probes more effectively than most other systems. There are numerous ways of finding such localized areas of dysfunction, as witness the methods advocated by Travell, Pruden, Nimmo as described in this chapter and others. However, many practitioners in the United Kingdom and United States have come to the conclusion that few other forms of trigger point assessment measure up to Lief's original methods in terms of ease of application, economy of time and effort, and efficiency of result.

Lief advocated the following of the exact same sequence of contacts on each occasion, whether assessing or treating, the difference between these modes being merely one of repetition of the strokes, with some degree of added pressure when treating. Lief's recommendation did not, however, mean that the same treatment was given each time, for the essence of NMT is that the pressure applied, both in diagnosis and in therapy is *variable*, and that this variability is determined by the tissues themselves. Thus while repetition of a diagnostic or therapeutic stroke might appear identical to its predecessor, it would differ depending upon the state of the tissues it was being taken through. This concept will become clearer as we progress.

A light lubricant is always used in NMT, to avoid skin drag; the main contact is made with the tip of the thumb(s) – more precisely the medial aspect of the tip, as a rule. In some regions the tip of the index or middle finger are used instead, as these allow easier access for insertion between the ribs for assessment (or treatment) of, for example, intercostal

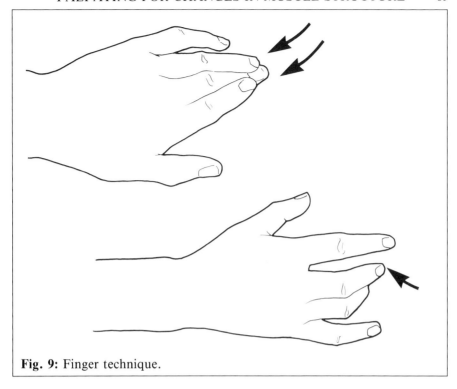

Fig. 9: Finger technique.

musculature. This 'finger contact' is identical with that suggested in *'bindegewebsmassage'* except that in the German system no lubricant is used.

Practitioner posture and positioning are important when applying NMT, as the correct application of forces reduces dramatically the energy expended, and the time taken to perform the assessment/treatment. It is suggested that the examination table should be of a height which allows the therapist to be able to stand erect, legs separated for ease of weight transference, with the assessing arm straight at the elbow. This allows the practitioner's body-weight to be transferred down the extended arm through the thumb, imparting any degree of force required – from extremely light to quite substantial – simply by leaning on the arm. (This presents a problem for a small number of practitioners whose thumbs are too flexible. A solution is for them to use only the finger contact described below.)

Weight transference from back to leading leg, with knees slightly flexed, is a sound way of controlling accurately the degree of pressure being applied while saving energy. It is important that the fingers of the assessing treating hand act as a fulcrum, and that they lie at the front of the contact, allowing the stroke made by the thumb to run across the palm of the hand, towards the ring or small finger as the stroke progresses.

This approach produces numerous benefits, the most important being control. Were the thumb merely pushed along through the tissues it

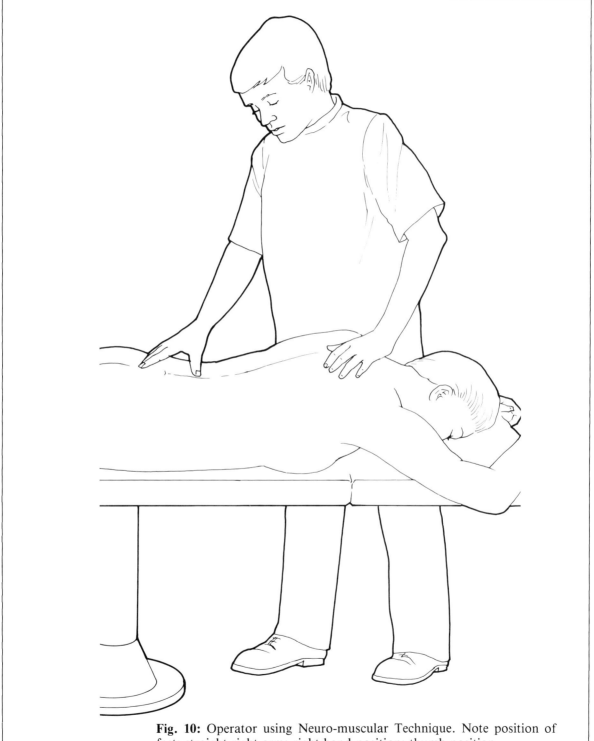

Fig. 10: Operator using Neuro-muscular Technique. Note position of feet; straight right arm; right hand position; thumb position.

would lack the delicacy of fine control which Lief's NMT demands. The finger/fulcrum remains stationary as the thumb draws intelligently towards it. Each stroke, whether it be diagnostic or therapeutic, extends for approximately 1.5–2 inches before the thumb ceases its motion, at which time the fulcrum fingers can be moved further ahead in the direction the thumb needs to travel. The thumb stroke continues, feeling and searching through the tissues.

Another vital ingredient, indeed the very essence of the thumb contact, is its application of variable pressure (diagnostic poundage is in ounces initially) which allows it to insinuate and tease its way through whatever fibrous, indurated or contracted structures it meets.

The degree of resistance or obstruction presented by the tissues determines the degree of effort required. Thus, in heavily tensed tissues, several pounds of pressure may be needed for a subsequent diagnostic stroke. Tense, contracted or fibrous tissues are never simply overcome by force, as this would irritate, and add to dysfunction. Rather, the fibres are worked through, using substantial pressure at times, but in a constantly varying manner in which both angles of application of pressure, and degrees of pressure, are constantly altered to meet the particular demands of the tissues.

A degree of vibrational contact, as well as the variable pressure allows the stroke and the contact to have an 'intelligent' feel, and seldom risk traumatizing or bruising tissues even when heavy pressure is used. As in the advice quoted in previous chapters, it is a requirement of NMT palpation/assessment that the thumb tip be seen as an extension of the brain, that an intelligent quality be added to the mechanical nature of its travels over and through tissue. The patient picks this up rapidly and senses that the approach is not just a mechanical process but an intimate response to the needs of his/her pain or dysfunction. As in much palpation it is usual to suggest that NMT be applied with eyes closed. A 'nice hurt' is all that is usually complained of even when pressure is fairly deep.

It is usual to try to get the medial tip of the thumb to be the precise contact and as a rule this is achieved after a little practice, unless there is hypermobility of the thumb joints preventing a stable contact of this sort. Whether thumb or finger contact is used (see below for discussion on finger contact) it is of some importance, both in terms of energy conservation and ease of application of NMT, that the arm and even the hand which is doing the work remain relatively relaxed.

This may seem to be a contradiction in terms. However, it requires some emphasis; if the muscles of the forearm are tensed unduly, or if the fingers which form the fulcrum towards which the thumbs move are rigid, an inordinate amount of energy will be wasted, the arm will tire rapidly, control will diminish, and the 'feel' to the patient will be harsh rather than gentle. Perception will be dulled in the process unless a relatively relaxed state is maintained throughout.

The finger fulcrum does not grasp, or dig into, the tissues on which it rests. It merely alights and rests there, with a minimal contact, as the thumb travels towards it. Effort, if any is required in terms of added pressure, is achieved by shifting body weight through the almost straight arm, not by using arm or hand strength.

When a finger contact is used instead of the thumb (which always travels away from the practitioner in a controlled manner, towards the finger fulcrum at the end of the extended arm) the hand is drawn towards the operator's body, with the treating finger slightly hooked, as in the methods of *bindegewebsmassage*. This allows for control of the hand and the use of body weight in a different manner to that applied when the thumb is employed. The other major area where finger contact is useful, apart from the intercostal structures, is the lateral pelvic region. Indeed as the palpating hand is brought towards the operator, over a curved surface, its main usefulness will be perceived. By leaning backwards, weight on the back leg, and allowing the hooked finger to be pulled through the tissues, a moderate degree of counterweight from the patient's inertia can be utilized, increasing depth of penetration with minimal effort for the practitioner.

Standing on the side opposite that being treated the hooked finger – supported by its neighbouring digit if necessary – can be inserted deeply into the intercostal space or the lateral pelvic musculature, above the trochanter, and as the practitioner leans back and allows the weight of the patient to apply drag, the fingers are slowly drawn through these tissues, thus assessing the nature of dysfunction in this region (or of applying cross-fibre or inhibitory contacts, if these contacts are being used therapeutically rather than diagnostically).

The pattern of strokes which Lief and Chaitow evolved is the one which allows maximum access to potential dysfunction in the shortest time, and with least demand for altered position and wasted effort. These strokes are illustrated, together with the suggested operator foot positions for each region.

Diagnostic assessment involves one superficial and one moderately deep contact only. If treatment is decided on at that time then several more strokes, applied from varying angles, would be used to relax the structures, to stretch them, to inhibit contraction, or to deal with trigger points elicited in the examination phase. Trigger point treatment is possible by use of direct inhibitory pressure followed by stretching of the affected musculature. (This is fully described in *Soft Tissue Manipulation* and *Instant Pain Control* by the author.)

In assessing (or treating) joint dysfunction or problems involving the extremities, it is suggested that all the muscles associated with a joint receive NMT attention, to origins and insertions, and that the bellies of the muscles be assessed as well for trigger points and other dysfunction. In this way not only the apparently affected joint receives attention but, at the very least, the ones above and below it. A full spinal assessment should be accomplished in 12 to 15 minutes with ease, once NMT is mastered. (Treatment of those areas which demand extra attention would add perhaps another 5 to 10 minutes.)

It is suggested that every patient receive full spinal and abdominal (including thoracic) neuromuscular assessment at least once at the outset of any programme, and that this should be repeated periodically to assess changes brought about by whatever treatment is decided upon. It is of course not necessary to do a full assessment at each visit and a diagnostic assessment of a localized region, accompanied by other diagnostic modalities and methods might be all that is necessary. By following a pattern which does not vary in its assessment of the regions illustrated, and most importantly by *recording whatever findings there are each time*, a clear individual pattern of dysfunction and localized structural changes can be established for each patient, and progress or lack of it readily noted.

With effective use of NMT, not only would localized, discrete, 'points' be discovered, but also patterns of stress bands, altered soft tissue mechanics, contractions and shortenings. Beal's rigid paraspinal tissues (see p.64) would be readily identified, as would the difference between changes resulting from viscerosomatic activity and localized dysfunction, as described by Magoun earlier in this chapter. NMT, in its therapeutic mode, has proved itself as an adjunct to manipulation, as well as often being able to obviate the need for other soft tissue, or osseous approaches. Even if only the diagnostic approach is adopted the patient will still have had 'a treatment', and will usually report marked benefits.

Is the term neuromuscular technique accurate? Knowledge of the function of the neural 'reporting' stations such as the various components of the muscle spindle, and Golgi tendon organs, has allowed us to understand how NMT achieves its results. When used near origins and insertions, the load detectors – the Golgi tendon organs – are clearly receiving mechanical input, especially if the direction of the stroke is towards the belly of the muscle. The effect of any degree of pressure away from the origin and insertion, towards the belly, would be initially to increase tone, and if sustained would produce reflex relaxation of the muscle.

If pressure is away from the belly of the muscle, near both the origin and insertion simultaneously, there will be a tendency for muscle to lose tone. The spindle registers length of muscle and rate of change of that length, and pressure via NMT would alter length locally, as well as having an inhibitory effect on neural discharge. Pressure inhibition of neural discharge is the main NMT contribution to trigger point treatment. The overall effect of NMT via neural mediation is one in which reduced tone is created in hypertonic structures, over and above the purely mechanical effects introduced by stretching, friction and drainage of fluids and toxic wastes.

Many hours of patient NMT work are required before the degree of sensitivity which allows the smallest local area of dysfunction to be identified is achieved. It is this idea of optimum palpatory literacy which should be the objective of those who utilize NMT.

Exercise 5. Begin to practise NMT by concentrating on body

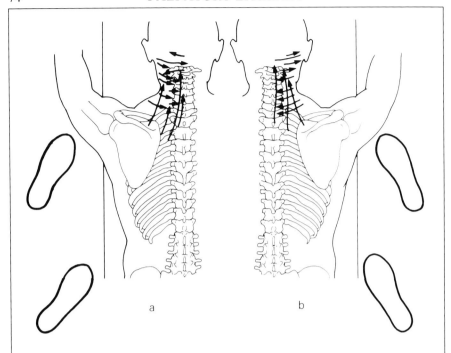

a   b

Fig. 11: Neuro-muscular Technique. Illustrating position of operator and lines of application.

position. Make sure your treatment surface is of a height which will allow you to stand in the manner illustrated and described, without hunching or stretching unduly. This position must allow a straight arm position (when the thumb contact is being used) and the ability to transfer weight to increase pressure without arm muscle activity being employed.

After applying a light lubricant, position yourself and place the hand according to the illustration and description, fingers acting as a fulcrum, thumb (medial tip) feeling through the tissues, slowly and with variable pressure.

Practise this, in no particular sequence of strokes, until the mechanics of the body-arm-hand-thumb positions are comfortable and require no thought.

Exercise 6. Choose an illustrated NMT sequence (d is ideal) and follow the strokes precisely as illustrated (although direction of strokes need not follow arrow directions). Chart any findings you make – tender areas, stress bands, contracted fibres, trigger points and so on. If TPs are found, note target area as well.

In this sequence there are intercostal strokes illustrated. Use the hooked finger contact to search these regions. Standing on left side of patient to assess right intercostals. Again note any findings.

Work slowly and try to follow the descriptions given above of the

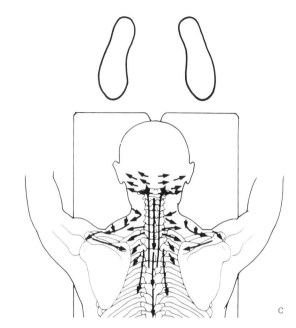

Fig. 11: Neuro-muscular Technique. Illustrating position of operator and lines of application.

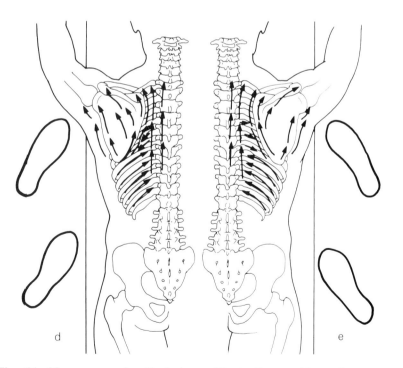

Fig. 11: Neuro-muscular Technique. Illustrating position of operator and lines of application.

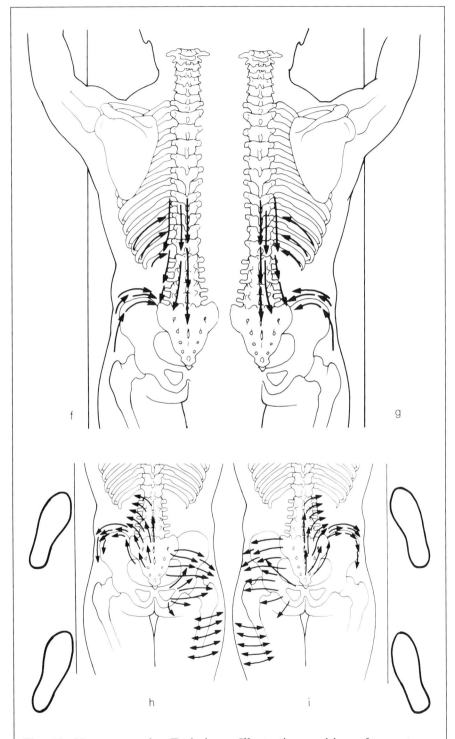

Fig. 11: Neuro-muscular Technique. Illustrating position of operator and lines of application.

way the thumb insinuates its way through the tissues, never overwhelming them, never gouging or pushing unfeelingly. Allow your palpating contact to be your eyes. Work with your eyes closed.

This sequence should take at least 15 minutes at first, reducing with practice to 3–4 minutes.

Exercise 7. Practice the abdominal/lower rib cage sequence as illustrated. Use lighter contacts than would have been appropriate for paraspinal musculature. See what soft tissue changes you can discover in these tissues, especially near origins and insertions, below the thoracic cage, near the pelvic and pubic insertions. If there are scars search diligently around these for sensitive and tight structures. For greater guidance as to this and other NMT sequences reference should be made to *Soft Tissue Manipulation*.

An abdominal NMT assessment should be achieved inside 15 minutes at first, with this reducing to 7–8 minutes once you are efficient with NMT.

Exercise 8. Work your way through the individually illustrated segments of the spinal NMT assessment, several times each, and then put them all together, doing a full spinal assessment, charting

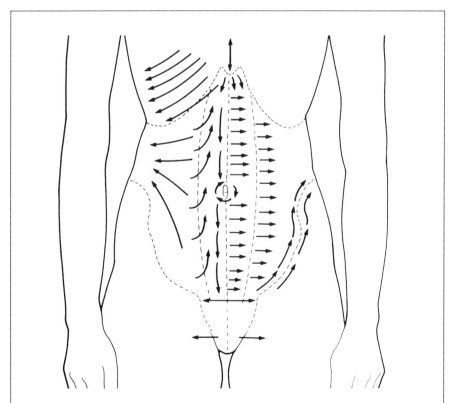

Fig. 12: Neuro-muscular general abdominal technique. Lines of application.

everything you find. At first this will take up to an hour. With practice it can be effectively and thoroughly done in 15 minutes.

Jones' Tender Points and Their Significance

Lawrence Jones described the evolution of his therapeutic methods, which partly depend upon identification of 'tender' points which are found in the proximity of joints which have been stressed, strained or traumatized, ('Strain/Counterstrain', *Academy of Applied Osteopathy*, Colorado Springs, 1981). These are identified, according to Dvorak and Dvorak, as 'swollen, flat regions in specific parts of the body'.

They are located in deep muscle, often in musculature which lies opposite (i.e., in the antagonist) to that which was stressed at the time of the strain or trauma. Thus in spinal problems resulting from a flexion strain in which back pain was complained of, for example, the appropriate 'tender' point would be found on the anterior surface of the body. It would itself be exquisitely sensitive on palpation, but painless otherwise. Once identified the points are used to position the area/body so that the palpated pain disappears or reduces substantially. Tissue tension usually eases at the same time and if held for some 90 seconds there is often a resolution of the dysfunction which resulted from the trauma.

This method is fully explained in Jones' book, and a modified version is described in my own *Soft Tissue Manipulation*. The reason for its inclusion in this survey is that awareness of its principles helps the therapist account for unexplained, and previously unreported sensitive areas uncovered during palpation, whether or not Jones' methods of treatment are then used. This knowledge can also be used to guide the therapist to the appropriate tissues (i.e., those tissues opposite the stretched tissues) in order to search for 'tender' points which might have resulted from acute or chronic strain on a joint or soft tissue area.

Such points are in all ways similar to Ah Shi points (spontaneously tender points) as reported in Traditional Chinese Medicine (TCM) for several thousands of years. In TCM, however, they are not used in the manner described above, but are considered to be amenable to acupuncture or acupressure methods for as long as they remain sensitive. These points are seldom also trigger points in that they do not refer pain to a distant target, but rather hurt locally.

Exercise 9. Palpate the tissues opposite those effectively stretched during a joint or spinal trauma or strain. These should be in an area not complained of as being painful. A localized very tender area in such tissue is a Jones tender point. Palpate this as you position the joint or area in such a way as to remove the tenderness from the palpated point. This usually involves some degree of increased slack in the palpated tissues. Hold this for 90 seconds and then slowly return to a neutral position and repalpate. Has the tenderness reduced, vanished? It should, and the joint should feel more normal. Try this a number of times until the concept becomes imprinted.

Travell and Simons' definition of Trigger Points (TP)

Travell and Simons', medical pioneers of our understanding of trigger points, describe specific characteristics which identify them from other myofascial changes:

1. A TP which is active causes pain to be referred to a predictable site and it is rarely located where the patient complains of pain.

2. There will be taut fibres (palpable bands) in the muscles which house TPs. Tension on such a band (stretching the muscle actively or passively) will refer pain to the target area.

3. There will be a palpable ropiness or nodularity in muscles which house TPs, and the muscle will have a reduction in its full range of motion.

4. A TP will be found at the site of the most sensitivity/tenderness in any taut band of muscle fibres.

5. If the tissue housing the TP is 'rolled' briskly by fingers or thumb (called 'snapping palpation' by Travell and Simons) so that there is a sudden change of pressure on it, a 'twitch' response* is observed. This, they claim, is unequivocal evidence of TP activity, latent or active.

6. Sustained digital pressure on the TP (or insertion into it of a needle) usually reproduces the referred pain pattern for which it is responsible.

Other autonomic phenomena may also be evoked, other than pain.

Dr Janet Travell maintains that the high intensity of nerve impulses from an active trigger point can produce, by reflex, vasoconstriction, cutting down the blood supply to specific areas of the brain, spinal cord and nervous system, thus producing any of a wide range of symptoms capable of affecting almost any part of the body. Among symptoms reported by Dr Travell, and others, are the following, all as a direct result of trigger point activity (as proved by their disappearance when the triggers were dealt with):

- pain
- numbness
- itching
- over-sensitivity to normal stimuli
- spasm
- twitching
- weakness and trembling of muscles
- over- or under-secretion of glands
- localized coldness
- paleness
- redness of tissues
- menopausal hot flashes
- altered texture of skin (very oily, very dry)
- increased sweat production

---

* Travell and Simons describe this so-called 'jump' sign as follows. The most sensitive part of the affected muscle is seen to shorten visibly when the relaxed muscle is passively stretched, if the firm band of the affected muscle is briskly 'snapped' by the palpating finger at the same time.

In triggers found in the abdominal and thoracic muscles:
- halitosis (bad breath)
- heartburn
- vomiting
- distension
- nervous diarrhoea and constipation, disordered vision, respiratory symptoms and skin sensitivity.

Travell also reports symptoms of 'hysteria' which disappear with successful trigger point work.

It must not be forgotten that trigger points, while causing symptoms themselves, are also caused by something else. Unless those causes are eliminated they will return, even if treatment eliminates them temporarily. Often new trigger points develop in target areas (reference zone); these are known as 'satellite' triggers. These require attention, just as much as their 'parent' trigger points do.

> **Exercise 10.** Find a trigger point using NMT (or any other method) and then go through the Simons/Travell guidelines to ensure it fills all requirements (other than inserting a needle into it, unless you are licensed to do so).

Raymond Nimmo's Assessment Plan for TPs

Raymond Nimmo D.C. developed a system which he called 'receptor-tonus' which systematically uncovered trigger points and then 'deactivated' them by inhibitory pressure, followed by stretching of the muscles involved if they were hypertonic, or strengthening if they were hypotonic. He also applied himself to what he termed 'noxious' points in ligaments. He diagnosed all noxious points by their sensitivity, claiming that, 'properly' applied pressure would elicit painful points in all hypertonic and hypotonic muscles.

He summarized his approach with: 'We have three things with which to deal, to wit: noxious or trigger points, ligament and tonus.' His method of identification of trigger or noxious points can be understood if we examine the following quote from his lecture notes (1966) which covers examination of the sub-scapular area for trigger points affecting the shoulder:

> Look about $2\frac{1}{2}$ inches to left of spinous processes on a level with the lower scapula border. Let the fingers glide along until a slight difference is found in the small muscles. If such a point is sensitive it should be treated.

After describing his method for dealing with the trigger (5 seconds sustained pressure, repeated if necessary) he continues:

> After holding pressure on a point, say on the level of the lower scapula border, move in a straight line upwards along the internal margin of the scapula about one inch. Here, usually, another point may be found. Treat it in the same manner and move upward about another inch and look for another point.

Nimmo states that 90 per cent of all patients will have trigger points in one of these sites. Referred pain will be to shoulder or head from these. He continues by suggesting the practitioner search the body in the following sites, where the given percentage will demonstrate active, sensitive, 'noxious' points. Only sensitive points are treated, never non-painful ones:

1. Superior angle of scapula, on tendon of *levator scapulae*. This refers to head, face, neck and shoulders: 90 per cent incidence reported.

2. Between and on the ribs, between the transverse processes and around rib heads. Triggers here indicate an imbalance between *paraspinal musculature* due to Davis' Law which states: 'if hypertonus exists on one side, tonus is released on the other side'. Affects most people.

3. Inferior angle of scapula, on inner insertions of *infraspinatus*. Also along inner border until spine of scapula is reached, working outwards until insertion of infraspinatus on humerus is palpated. 'After this, search the space toward the lateral edge of the scapula, letting thumb fall off outwardly, then flipping it back on, pressing partly against *infraspinatus* and partly against fascia beneath and also on *teres minor*. Here is a favourite place for trouble. It will usually refer to the back of the arms and to the 4th and 5th fingers. Upper *infraspinatus* refers to front of shoulders.' 90 per cent of patients have triggers here.

4. Press on internal aspect of *supraspinatus* moving laterally towards its insertion. Triggers here are a common cause of 'tired' shoulders. A 40 per cent incidence of triggers at this site is reported.

5. Search outer border of scapula for *teres major* points. Triggers are common if patient cannot raise arm behind back. 60 per cent of patients were found by Nimmo to have triggers in these muscles.

6. *Trapezius* is searched by squeezing it between fingers and thumb, moving slowly from shoulder region towards spine until triggers are found. Pain refers to mastoid area or to forehead. Very common – 90 per cent.

7. Pressure (firm, says Nimmo) on superior border of sacrum, between iliac spine and sacral spinous process produces pressure on *SI ligament*. Move contact superiorly and inferiorly searching for sensitivity. Triggers here are involved in all low back syndromes and 50 per cent of all patients according to Nimmo. As in all descriptions given it is suggested that you search both sides.

8. Press just superiorly to sacral base adjacent to spine medial to PSIS. This is *iliolumbar ligament*. Heavy pressure is required to find triggers which are involved in most low back problems. Search both sides. (90 per cent incidence reported.)

9. Hook thumb under *sacrosciatic* and *sacrotuberous* ligaments medial and inferior to ischial tuborosity, lifting and stretching laterally if painful. Nimmo reports a 30 per cent incidence of triggers in these sites.

Note: Nimmo used a palm-held rubber-tipped wooden T-bar, in order to apply pressure to areas requiring high poundage such as iliolumbar ligament.

10. Medial pressure is applied by the thumb to lateral border of *quadratus lumborum* avoiding pressure on tips of transverse processes starting below last rib down to pelvic rim. A 'gummy' feel will be noted if contracture exists (plus sensitivity) in contrast to 'resilient, homogenous feel' of normal muscle. Often associated with low back problems. If *latissimus dorsi* is also involved, pain may radiate to shoulder or arm, 80 per cent of patients show trigger activity in these muscles, based on Nimmo's research.

11. Search area below posterior aspect of ilia for noxious points associated with *gluteal muscles* generally.

12. Search central region of belly of *gluteus medius* for triggers which can produce sciatic-type pain. (90 per cent incidence).

13. Search midway between trochanters and superior crest of ilium, in central portion of *gluteus minimus* where trigger affecting lateral aspect of leg or foot, or duplicating sciatic-type pain, is common. This also has a 90 per cent incidence of triggers, as opposed to *gluteus maximus*, which produces active triggers in only 4 per cent of patients.

14. The point of intersection where imaginary lines drawn from the PSIS and the trochanter, and the ischium and the ASIS, meet, is the access point for contact with the insertion of the *piriformis* muscle. If the line from the ASIS is taken to the coccyx the intersection is over the belly of piriformis. These two points should be palpated, if sensitivity is noted the muscle requires treatment. Sciatic distribution to the knee is a common referred symptom. A 40 per cent incidence of triggers is reported by Nimmo.

15. *Hamstring* trigger points lie about a hand's width above the knee joint in about 20 per cent of patients.

16. Trigger points in *abductor magnus* muscles lie close to its origins and insertions, notably near the tendinous insertion, and close to the ischium.

17. The area *posterior* to the *tibia* is a site for trigger points relating to calf pain. 90 per cent of patients display triggers here according to Nimmo.

18. Triggers abound in the region of the *external malleolus*, especially if recurrent ankle strains have occurred.

19. With patient side-lying and operator standing facing patient at chest level, reach across with cephalid hand to ease scapula into maximum abduction while thumb of the caudad hand is inserted under scapula to try to contact *seratus magnus* and *subscapularis* muscles (both have 90 per cent incidence of triggers). Careful probing allows contact with triggers and restrictions, which occur in 90 per cent of individuals.

20. Search for triggers in the *upper cervical* muscles with patient face upwards and operator's thumb applying pressure against these

muscles, medially and upwards (to ceiling) along length of lamina groove from occiput to base of neck, 90 per cent of patients have triggers in these muscles.

21. Same position, right hand under and cupping lower neck, thumb anterior to trapezius fibres, rotate head to right allowing hand to slowly glide towards floor. Thumb can descend into 'pocket' created by the head position. When thumb has reached as far as possible, pressure with it towards the opposite nipple allows contact to be made with insertion of *splenius capitus* muscle (around 2nd thoracic vertebra). Referred pain to base of neck is common symptom. Again, 90 per cent of people have triggers here.

22. Standing at head of patient place right thumb just superior to clavicle, lateral to outer margin of sternomastoid, flex neck by raising head with other hand allowing right thumb to enter area below clavicle over attachment of *anterior scalene* muscle. Patient's head is turned right bringing scalene directly under thumb. Pressure laterally with thumb finds triggers located here, a common (90 per cent) finding.

23. *Anterior cervical* muscles are palpated for changes and trigger points by facing seated patient and inserting thumbs under jawline, to contact anterior surface of upper transverse processes. Gliding thumbs inferiorly allows contact with *longus capitus*, *coli* and so on, (70 per cent trigger point incidence). Care is required as to degree of pressure and time spent in the region of carotid body.

24. *Sternomastoid* palpation is performed with patient face upwards head turned towards side being assessed. Contact is by 'squeezing' between finger(s) and thumb as direct pressure is avoided in this muscle (as in scalene, apart from its insertions).

25. Triggers lying in *masseter* and *external pterygoid* muscles are found with operator sitting at head of supine patient. Problems here relate to TMJ dysfunction, tinnitus and salivary gland dysfunction.

26. Functional disturbances of the eyes may stem from active triggers in *temporalis* muscle, which is palpated from same position as 25.

27. Standing to side of supine patient grasp wrist with cephalid hand and abduct the arm; other hand contacts coracoid process and thumb contact glides towards sternum assessing *subclavius* muscle. A similar stroke from coracoid process towards xyphoid assesses *pectoralis minor* (Nimmo reports a 90 per cent incidence of triggers in both muscles, only 10 per cent in *pectoralis major*).

28. Thumb pressure should be applied to *biceps tendon* insertion for a distance of an inch or so below its insertion in search of a trigger which would relate to shoulder problems (90 per cent incidence).

29. Trigger points are found on the sternum in the *rudimentary sternalis* muscle (40 per cent incidence of triggers) as well as in *cartilaginous attachments* of ribs on sternum.

30. With supine patient, knees flexed, contact is flat of hand (fingers more than palm) with other hand on top of it, applying pressure from just inferior to rib margins, going under these as far as possible to

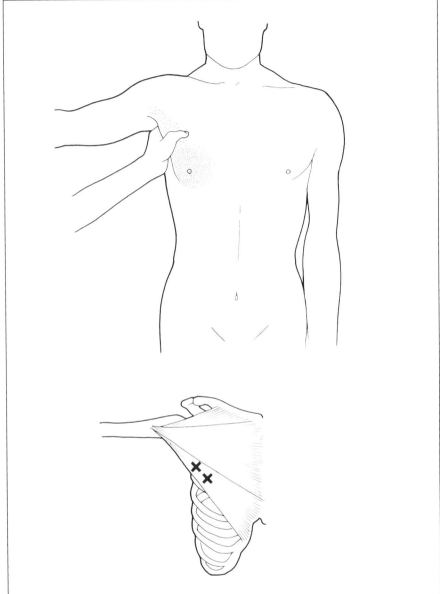

Fig. 13: Illustrating trigger points and target area (shaded) in pectoralis major muscle (sternocostal fibres) and ideal palpation method in this area (as well as trapezius, sternomastoid and scalenes).

a) Pincer palpation of trigger points in the sternocostal fibres of the pectoralis major muscle.

b) Referred pain patterns (black) and trigger points (xs) in the left pectoralis major muscle. Solid area shows essential areas of referred pain, and stippled area shows the spillover pain areas. The lateral free margin of the muscle, which includes fibres of the costal and abdominal sections that form the anterior axillary fold.

approach triggers lying in *upper abdominal* musculature (90 per cent). Finger pads are stroked in a series of movements from the most superior point reached under the ribs, towards the umbilicus. Tight bands will be felt in which triggers reside.

31. *Serratus magnus* is searched with flat of hand stretching it towards its attachments (90 per cent incidence).

32. Patient same position. Operator standing on side opposite that to be assessed and starting some 3 inches below umbilicus on a line from it to the ASIS, a firm flat hand contact is made; this is taken inferior and then medial allowing contact to be made *anterior to 4 and 5th lumbar vertebrae* (site of hypogastric plexus and ganglionated cord). This is likely to be an area of referred sensitivity (upwards to chest) in 70 per cent of patients. This contact could be avoided in the elderly, the obese, or patients with anneurisms or sclerotic aortas.

33. Patient in same position, operator standing on side to be examined, place fingerpads just superior to ASIS, pressing towards floor and then towards feet allow access to occur under the pelvic crest, to contact *iliacus* muscle. A gliding contact followed by flexing of the contact fingers allows searching of this area for triggers (90 per cent).

34. Access to the *psoas* muscle is suggested from lateral margin of rectus abdominus allowing finger contact to pass under the sigmoid on the left and under the caecum on the right. This accesses the belly of psoas in non-obese patients. Another access is directly towards the spine from the midline (patient with flexed knees) some 3 inches below umbilicus. On approaching the spine (denser feel) fingerpad contact slides laterally over body of lumbar vertebrae (2, 3 or 4) to side opposite. This will contact origin of psoas, a common site for triggers (50–70 per cent).

35. *Abductor longus* and *pectineus* can be contacted with patient in same position as thumbs glide along abductor towards pubic attachment and then laterally to contact pectineus. 50 per cent of patients have triggers in this muscle.

36. *Quadriceps* can be contacted and searched with thumbs, heel of hand or fingers, with patient supine. Triggers abound in both *rectus femoris* (90 per cent incidence) and the *Vasti* (70 per cent).

37. *Tensor fascia lata* is best contacted with patient side-lying, affected leg straight, supported by flexed other leg. Triggers here can produce sciatic-type pain (70 per cent).

38. *Gracilis* attachment into the knee region (via its tendon) is a major trigger site (90 per cent). The muscle itself should be assessed from tibial attachment to the pubis.

39. *Anterior tibialis* muscle may rarely contain triggers affecting feet or toes.

Exercise 11. Choose several of Nimmo's suggested targets, for example as in description 1 or 2, and see whether you can find active trigger points by following his instructions.

Compare this approach with that suggested in the description of Lief's NMT assessment. Many find a combination of these approaches is ideal.

Lewit's View of Trigger Point Significance

Karel Lewit M.D. suggests that, apart from their local significance in terms of pain, and their influence on target areas, trigger points can have a clinical significance in the links they have with certain pathology. For example:

- Triggers in the thigh adductors indicate hip pathology
- Triggers in iliacus indicate lesions of segments L5/S1 (coccyx)
- Triggers in piriformis indicate lesions of segment L4/5 (coccyx)
- Triggers in rectus femoris indicate lesions of L3/4 (hip)
- Triggers in psoas indicate lesions of thoracolumbar junction (T10-L1)
- Triggers in erector spinae muscles indicate lesions of corresponding spinal level
- Triggers in rectus abdominis indicate problems at xyphoid, pubis or low back
- Triggers in pectoralis indicate problems of upper ribs or thoracic viscera
- Triggers in subscapularis common in 'frozen shoulder'
- Triggers in middle trapezius indicate radicular syndrome of the upper extremity
- Triggers in upper trapezius indicate cervical lesion
- Triggers in sternomastoid indicate lesion of CO/1 and C2/3
- Triggers in masticatory muscles relate to headache and facial pain.

Lewit makes similar connections between periosteal pain points and specific functional or structural pathology.

Periosteal Pain Points (PPP)

As tonus increases and becomes chronically entrenched, leading to changes in the structure of the soft tissues, with increased fibrous and decreased elastic content becoming palpably apparent, so do stresses build up on the tendons and their osseous insertions into the periosteum. Many are characteristic of certain lesions, making them useful as diagnostic aids.

The feel of periosteal pain points varies but a frequently palpated common feature is of a sensitive 'soft bump' at the point of attachment of tendons and ligaments. This is often observed on spinous processes where one side is tender, relating to tension or spasm in the muscles on that side, which also prevents easy rotation of the body of that vertebrae to that side. Intervertebral joints can be palpated directly in some areas, for example the cervical joints are accessible when the patient is supine. Greater pressure is required through paraspinal tissues with the patient prone for access to other spinal joints (for example, using NMT approaches as described above).

Many extremity joints are available for direct palpation. The hip can be reached via the groin if care is taken. Acromioclavicular and sternoclavicular joints are easily accessed as is the TMJ anterior to the tragus.

Some PPP and their Significance According to Lewit

- A PPP sited at the head of the metatarsals indicates metatarsalgia (flat foot)
- A calcaneal spur (a classical PPP) indicates tension in the plantar aponeurosis
- A PPP sited at the tubercle of the tibia indicates tension in the long adductors, possibly a hip lesion
- A PPP sited at the attachments of the collateral knee ligaments indicates a lesion of the corresponding meniscus
- A PPP sited at the fibula head indicates tension in the biceps femoris or restriction of the head of the fibula
- A PPP sited on the PSIS is common but has no specific indication
- A PPP sited at lateral aspect of symphysis pubis indicates tension in the adductors, SI joint restriction or a hip lesion
- A PPP sited on the coccyx indicates tension in gluteus maximus, levator ani or piriformis
- A PPP sited on the iliac crest indicates gluteus medius or quadratus lumborum tension of dysfunction at thoracolumbar junction
- A PPP sited at the greater trochanter indicates tension in the abductors or a hip lesion
- A PPP sited on T5/6 spinous process indicates a lesion of the lower cervical spine
- A PPP sited on spinous process of C2 indicates a lesion at C1/2 or C2/3 or tension in levator scapulae
- A PPP sited on the xyphoid process indicates tension in rectus abdominis or 6, 7 or 8th rib dysfunction
- A PPP sited on the ribs in the mammary or axillary line indicates tension in pectoralis attachments or a visceral disorder
- A PPP sited at sternocostal junction of upper ribs indicates tension in the scalene muscles
- A PPP sited on the sternum, close to the clavicle indicates tension in sternomastoid muscle
- A PPP sited on the transverse process of the atlas indicates a lesion of the atlas/occiput segment or tension in either rectus capitis laterales or sternomastoid
- A PPP sited on the styloid process of the radius indicates an elbow lesion
- A PPP sited on the epicondyles indicates elbow lesion or tension in muscles attaching to epicondyles
- A PPP sited at attachment of the deltoid indicates a scapulohumeral joint lesion
- A PPP sited on the condyle of the mandible indicates a TMJ lesion or tension in the masticatory muscles

Exercise 12. Work your way through the PPP points as described above, and see how many are present as sensitive, palpable, structures in the patient/model. Try to compare the possibly involved soft tissues as indicated in the descriptions above. Are they indeed involved? Prove the usefulness of making the connection between a PPP and the soft tissue dysfunction which caused it.

Chapman's Neurolymphatic Reflex Points

We have seen that some viscerosomatic reflex activity is associated with facilitated spinal segment, and that another form of localized facilitation can be devastatingly involved in soft tissue dysfunction: the ubiquitous trigger point. The associated changes are palpable both via the skin and through the soft tissue changes they involve. Other soft tissue changes which might be picked up during palpation are Jones' tender points, which are associated with joint strain or trauma. We now need to examine, albeit briefly, another reflex system which is assessed by careful palpation.

In the 1930s osteopathic physician Frank Chapman, and subsequently his brother-in-law Charles Owens D.O., charted a group of palpable reflex changes which they termed neurolymphatic reflexes. In Owens' book on this topic (*An Endocrine Interpretation of Chapman's Reflexes*) the palpable changes, consistently associated with the same viscera which are found in the fascia, are described thus:

> These little tissue changes (gangliform contractions) are located anteriorly in the intercostal spaces near the sternum. They may vary in size from one-half the size of a BB shot, to that of a small bean, and occasionally are multiple. This type of change is apparent in some of the reflexes found on the pelvis, but the ones found on the lower extremity (colon, broad ligament and prostate) vary in character. Here there may be areas of 'amorphous shotty plaques' or 'stringy masses'.

The variations in texture result, according to these researchers, from a combination of both the nature and severity of the visceral involvement and the constitution of the patient. The degree of tenderness noted on palpation differentiates these from what the authors term 'fat globules'. In some areas, such as in the rectus femoris muscle, reflexes (from suprarenal gland) have the feel of acute contraction. Posterior reflexes are found mainly between the spinous processes and the tips of the transverse processes, where they have more of an oedematous feel, and sometimes a 'stringy' nature on deeper palpation.

Beryl Arbuckle D.O. discussed Chapman's initial discovery of these reflexes in her fine collection *Selected Writings of Beryl Arbuckle*:

> Chapman found highly congested points in different regions of the fascia, and with certain very definite groupings he found to exist a definite entity of disease or, reversely, with a particular disease he always found a definite pattern in these regions. These findings led him to conclude that the states of hypercongestion were due to a lymph stasis, in viscus, or gland, which was manifested by soreness or tenderness at the distal ends of the spinal

nerves. To understand this reasoning one must have a knowledge of the lymphatic system, the autonomic nervous system, and the interrelation of the endocrine glands, and the embryologic segmentation of the body.

Note: It is suggested that Arbuckle's thoughts be kept in mind when the Erlinghauser's research into cerebrospinal fluid circulation through tubular connective tissue fibrils is discussed in Chapter 5. Arbuckle sites, in support of Chapman's concepts, the amazing research of Speransky (see *A Basis for the Theory of Medicine*) which demonstrated beyond doubt that CSF travels through the lymphatics to all areas of the body. This fact (now reinforced by Erlinghauser's work) combined with knowledge of the many nutrient substances carried by nerve axons – the end products (metabolites) of which re-enter the lymphatic system – strongly supports Chapman's concept of neurolymphatic reflexes. Charts and means of application of these reflexes are to be found in Owen's *An Endocrine Interpretation of Chapman's Reflexes* as well as in my text *Soft Tissue Manipulation*.

Arbuckle says, 'Trained, seeing, sensing, feeling fingers.... are able to ''open some of the windows and doors'' for the correction of perverted circulation of fluids.' How easy is it?

Owen says:

> You may not at first be able readily to locate the gangliform contractions with ease, but with practice you will acquire a readiness of tactile perception that will greatly facilitate your work. Do not use excessive pressure on either anterior or posterior (p.90-94).

The suggestion by Chapman, Owens and Arbuckle is that these points are only active – and therefore of use for treatment purposes – if both the anterior and posterior points of a pair are active, as evidenced by both of them being both palpable and sensitive. The degree of sensitivity of the anterior of the pair indicates the degree of associated lymphatic congestion.

The sequence suggested is to start by palpating the anterior reflexes. If any are found to be active by virtue of being easily palpable and sensitive, the pair of this reflex is then examined posteriorly. If this is also palpable and sensitive, treatment commences on the anterior reflex point.

Gentle rotary pressure is used in the treatment phase, dosage being determined by palpation. You should procure a decrease in oedema, dissolution of the gangliform contracture in the deep fascia, and subsidence of the tenderness in the anterior reflex areas. The actual time involved may be from 20 seconds to two minutes.

Rechecking for sensitivity is suggested by gentle palpation. This gives a strong indication of the success or otherwise of the effort thus far. Since these are reflex areas, the skin overlaying them would be subject to the influences discussed in Chapter 3. These points can therefore be found by looking for them specifically, once you have knowledge of their existence, or by skin stretching, or via a systematic soft tissue assessment, such as Lief advocated. If this system interests you spend

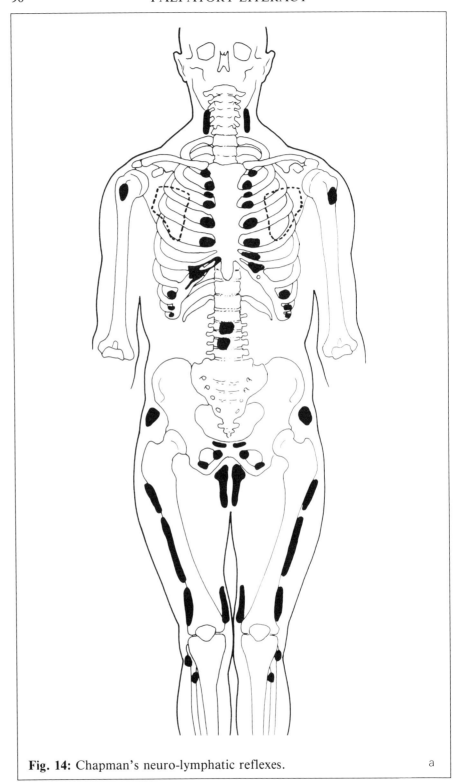

Fig. 14: Chapman's neuro-lymphatic reflexes.

a

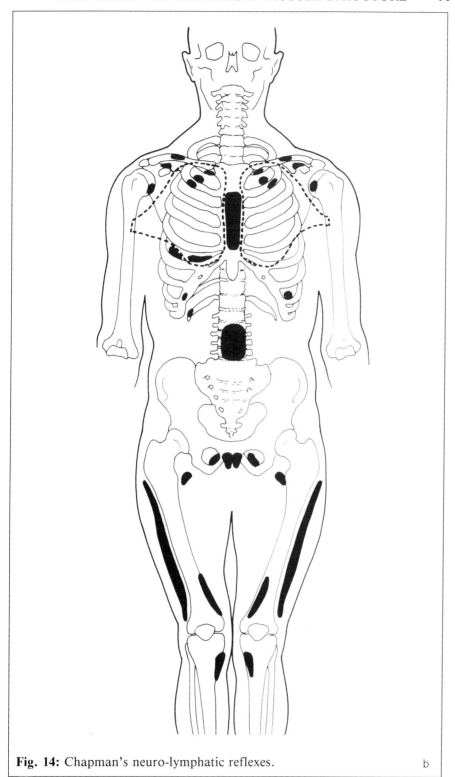

Fig. 14: Chapman's neuro-lymphatic reflexes.   b

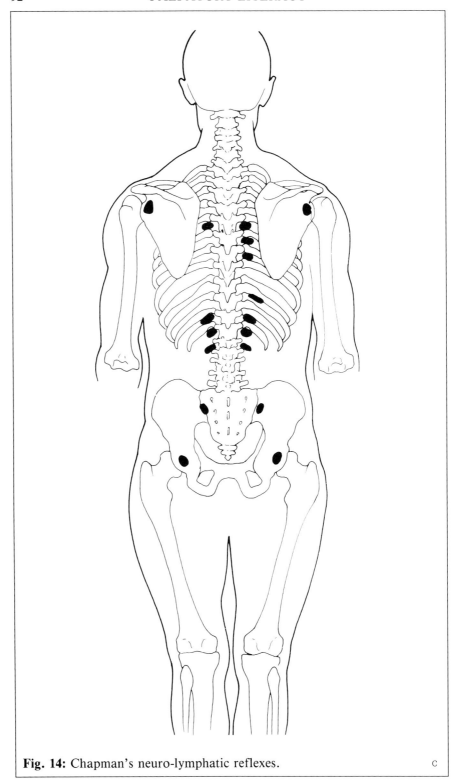

Fig. 14: Chapman's neuro-lymphatic reflexes.   c

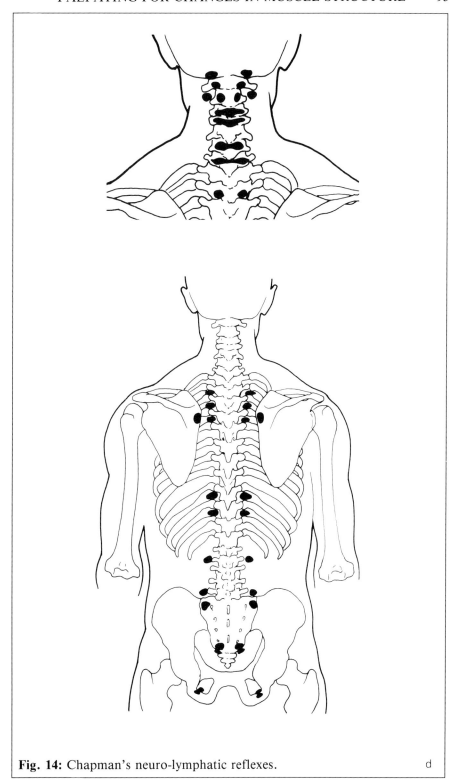

Fig. 14: Chapman's neuro-lymphatic reflexes.

d

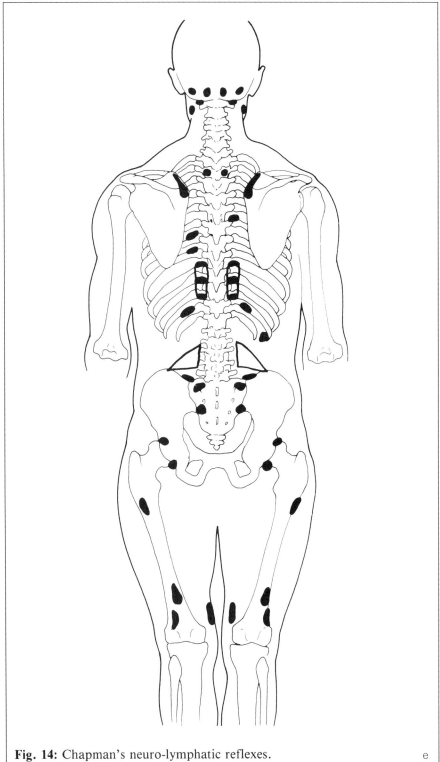

Fig. 14: Chapman's neuro-lymphatic reflexes.

e

some time palpating for pairs of neurolymphatic points as illustrated and described above.

Assessing Tight Postural Muscles

The final segment of this section will deal with a sequence in which short postural muscles may be identified.

Vladimir Janda M.D. in *Muscle Function Testing* confirms that postural muscles have a tendency to shorten, not only under pathological conditions but often under normal circumstances. Postural muscles are genetically older; they have different physiological and probably biochemical qualities compared with phasic muscles, which normally weaken and exhibit signs of inhibition in response to stress or pathology.

Most of the problems of the musculoskeletal system involve pain related to aspects of muscle shortening. Where weakness (lack of tone) is apparently a major element it will often be found that antagonists to these are shortened, reciprocally inhibiting their tone, and that prior to any effort to strengthen weak muscles, hypertonic antagonists should be dealt with by appropriate means, after which spontaneous toning occurs in the previously flaccid muscles. If tone is still inadequate then, and only then, should exercise and/or isotonic procedures be brought in.

We should, as part of comprehensive palpation, learn to assess short, tight muscles in a standardized manner. Janda suggests:

> To obtain a reliable evaluation the starting position, method of fixation and direction of movement must be observed carefully. The prime mover must not be exposed to external pressure. If possible the force exerted on the tested muscle must not work over two joints. The examiner performs at an even speed a slow movement that brakes slowly at the end of the range. To keep the stretch and the muscle irritability about equal the movement must not be jerky. Pressure or pull must always act in the required direction of movement. Muscle shortening can only be correctly evaluated if the joint range is not decreased as in a bony limitation or joint restriction.

See notes on pages 151–4 for descriptions of different end-feel characteristics.

It is in shortened muscles, as a rule, that reflex activity is noted. This takes the form of local dysfunction variously named as trigger points, tender points, zones of irritability, neurovascular and neurolymphatic reflexes. Localizing these is possible, via normal palpatory methods or as part of neuromuscular diagnostic treatment. Identification of tight muscles may be systematically carried out as described below. The following tests are derived from the work of Janda, Kendall and Boynton, and a variety of other sources.

Assessment of tight Gastrocnemius and/or soleus

Tests for Postural Muscle Shortening

1. Patient is supine with feet extending over edge of couch. For right leg examination operator's left hand grasps achilles tendon just above

heel, with no pressure on tendons. The heel lies in the palm of the hand, fingers curving round it. The right hand is placed so that the fingers rest on the dorsum of the foot (fingers rest all the time, do not apply a pulling stretch) with the thumb on the sole, lying along the lateral margin. This position is important as mistakes may involve placing the thumb too near the centre of the sole of the foot. Stretch is introduced by a pull on the heel with the left hand, while the right hand maintains the upward pressure via the thumb (along its entire length). The heel of the right hand prevents sideways movement of the foot.

A range should be achieved which takes the foot to a 90 degree angle to the leg. The leg must remain resting on the couch all the while and the left hand holding the heel must be placed so that it is an extension of the leg, not allowing an upward pull when stretch is introduced.

2. An alternative method is to have the patient seated on the couch, legs outstretched and to have him/her bend towards the toes with arms extended. If toe touching is possible, but toes are planter-flexed, then there is probably shortness of the gastrocnemius-soleus muscles.

Assessment of tight soleus

3. Method 1 assesses gastrocnemius and soleus. To assess soleus alone the same procedure is adopted with the knee passively flexed (over a cushion for example).

4. Patient is asked to squat, trunk slightly flexed, feet apart, so that the buttocks rest between the legs. It should be possible to go fully into this position with the heels flat on the floor. If not, and the heels rise from the floor as the squat is performed, soleus is shortened.

Assessment of shortness in Flexors of the Hip

5. Patient is supine with buttocks at end of couch, coccyx almost over the edge. The leg not being assessed is flexed as far as possible in order to tilt the pelvis posteriorly to flatten the lumbar curve against the couch. This leg is held (by patient and operator) in order to maintain this position of the pelvis. The leg to be tested should lie so that the upper leg is horizontal to the surface of the couch with the lower leg hanging down freely.

If the thigh cannot lie horizontal to the couch then it indicates a shortened iliopsoas muscle. Additional downward pressure on the distal thigh applied by the operator, should allow for extension at the hip, if it does not then the iliopsoas is very much shortened. (See also pp.85, 132, 187 for more on psoas assessment.)

If the lower leg cannot flex completely to hang vertically in this position, then there is a probable shortening of rectus femoris. If additional downward pressure on the lower third of the femur of the tested leg results in compensatory extension of the lower leg, at the knee, then rectus femoris is very short.

If both hip and knee are flexed as above (thigh unable to lie horizontal to surface of couch and lower leg unable to hang vertically) then both iliopsoas and rectus femoris are shortened.

If there is a marked lateral deviation of the patella, and a deep hollow groove is noted on the outer thigh, then tensor fascia lata is probably shortened. If additional pressure is applied on the lower third of the thigh of the tested leg, to take it slightly more into adduction, and this increases the hollow in the outer thigh over the iliobibial band then the tensor fascia lata is very short. (See also pp.85, 187 for more on TFL assessments.)

6. The patient is side-lying, tested leg uppermost. Lower leg is flexed and held to the couch. Upper leg is flexed at hip and knee and is abducted and extended by the operator, whose hand holds this leg at the ankle thus allowing the knee to fall into adduction, towards the couch. It will not do so if there is shortening of the iliotibial band, even if the patient is totally relaxed.

Assessment of Shortened Hamstrings (biceps, femoris, semitendinosus and Semimembranosis)

7. Patient is supine with legs outstretched. In order to assess tightness in the left leg hamstrings the right leg must be fixed to the couch by a downward pressure applied above the knee, avoiding the patella, by the operators cephalid hand. The operator is standing at the side of the leg to be tested, facing the couch. The lower leg is grasped with his/her caudad hand, keeping the knee of that leg in extension and resting the heel of that leg in the bend of the elbow to prevent lateral rotation of the leg. Range of movement should allow elevation of the leg to about 80 degrees.

8. If the hip flexors are shortened as assessed using the methods above (5), thus causing a forward tilt of the pelvis and stretch of the hamstrings, a modification of 7 is required.

The patient is supine with the leg not to be tested at the hip with the sole of the foot on the couch. This tilts the pelvis backwards and allows the lumbar curve to remain flat against the couch. All other aspects of 7 above are repeated as a test for short hamstrings is carried out.

9. As in 2 above. If the patient cannot reach the toes and the pelvis is relatively posteriorly tilted when patient is fully flexed, then the hamstrings are probably tight.

10. Toe touching may be possible but it may be observed that most of the flexion ability relates to exaggerated flexibility of the upper back muscles. Hamstrings may be shortened (as may low back muscles.)

11. If in this same procedure the patient can barely sit upright with legs extended, and is actually leaning backwards, then low back, hamstrings and gastroc-soleus are probably shortened.

In all these tests the knee of the tested leg must not flex at the knee.

12. Supine patient places leg to be tested so that operator (standing lateral to the leg, facing cephalid) can rest the foot of the straight leg in the crook of his/her couchside elbow. Non-tested leg is placed in

slight abduction with foot over the edge of the end of the couch. Operator's couchside hand rests on the anterolateral aspect of the tibia maintaining downward pressure to ensure constant extension of the lower leg. The other hand is in contact with the lateral thigh distal to the trochanter. Lateral rotation of the foot is prevented by its position against the operator's upper arm. The pelvis and untested leg should remain in position throughout and be fixed if possible. Abduction is introduced to its maximum. When limit is reached the knee is flexed and further abduction attempted.

Abduction should be possible to about 40 degrees. If there is an increase in abduction when the knee is flexed then it is assumed gracilis and biceps femoris (medial hamstrings) are shortened, their influence being removed by knee flexion. If there is no increase in range with knee flexed it can be assumed that pectinius and the abductors are shortened. Comparison of the two legs is needed to assess which has the greater range.

Testing for Shortness of Piriformis

13. When short the supine patient will display external rotation of the leg on the side of shortness as well as a shorter leg on that side. Patient is supine with tested leg flexed at hip and knee. Operator maintains pressure along long axis of flexed leg, at the knee, to fix pelvis. This leg is flexed, adducted and medially rotated using a contact on the medial aspect of the lower leg. Adduction/medial rotation will be limited and uncomfortable at the end of the range if piriformis is short. (See also pp.82, 190 for more on piriformis assessment.)

Assessment of Shortness in Quadratus Lumborum

14. Patient stands legs apart and sidebends, ensuring that this does not involve any flexion or rotation. The relative range of sidebending is compared to each side. Avoid any twisting of trunk, bending forward or back, and sideways movement of pelvis. Sliding the hand down the side of the leg is an ideal method. At maximum sidebending the upper shoulder should lie above the inter-gluteal line. This is not totally reliable as a means of assessment. (See also exercise 9 p.190.)

Assessment of Shortness in Paravertebral Muscles

15. Patient is seated on couch, legs extended, pelvis vertical. Flexion is introduced in order to approximate forehead to knees. An even curve should be observed and a distance of about 4 inches from the knees achieved by the forehead. No knee flexion should occur and the movement should be a spinal one, not involving pelvic tilting.

16. Patient sits at edge of couch, knees flexed and lower legs hanging over edge. Hamstrings are thus relaxed. Forward bending is introduced so that forehead approximates the knees. Pelvis is fixed. If bending of trunk is greater in this position than in 14, then there is probably tilting of the pelvis and shortened hamstring involvement.

During these assessments, areas of shortening in the spinal muscles may be observed; for example on forward bending a lordosis may be maintained in the lumbar spine, or flexion may be very limited even without such lordosis. There may be obvious overstretching of the upper back and relative tightness of the lower back. Generally 'flat' areas of the spine indicate local shortening of erector spinae group. There should be a uniform degree of flexion throughout.

Assessment of Thoraco-lumbar dysfunction
17. This important transition region is the only one in the spine in which two mobile structures meet, and dysfunction results in alteration of the quality of motion between the structures (upper and lower trunk-dorsal and lumbar spines). In dysfunction there is often a degree of spasm or tightness in the muscles which stabilize the region, notably psoas, erector spinae of the thoraco-lumbar region, often quadratus lumborum and rectus abdominus.

Symptomatic diagnosis of muscle involvement is possible as follows. Psoas involvement usually involves abdominal pain if severe and produces flexion of the hip and the typical antalgesic posture of lumbago. Erector spinae involvement produces low back pain at its caudal end of attachment and interscapular pain at its thoracic attachment (as far up as the mid-thoracic level).

Quadratus lumborum involvement causes lumbar pain and pain at the attachments on the iliac crest and lower ribs. Rectus abdominus contraction may mimic abdominal pain and result in pain at the attachments at the pubic symphysis and the xyphoid process as well as forward bending of the trunk and restricted ability to extend the spine. There is seldom pain at the site of the lesion in thoraco-lumbar dysfunction.

Assessment is by direct palpation of the various muscles for contraction and sensitivity.
18. Screening involves having the patient straddle the couch in a slightly flexed posture (slight kyphosis). Rotation in either direction enables segmental impairment to be observed as the spinous processes are monitored. Restriction of rotation is the most common characteristic. (See also p.187 for more on lumbo-dorsal junction dysfunction.)

Assessment of Shortness in Pectoralis Major
18. Patient supine lying with arms alongside the body and side to be tested near the edge of the couch. The tested arm is held at the mid-humeral level and is moved passively from the starting position upward and outward with the palm facing the ceiling. The upper arm should reach the horizontal plane and with additional pressure be able to increase its range of movement. It is possible in this position to palpate for tightened areas in the muscle. The upper arm will not reach the horizontal plane if there is such shortening. The location of the shortening is discovered by palpation. The thorax should be

stabilized during the raising of the arm so that no twisting of the thorax occurs and no increase in lordosis is noted. The humerus, not the forearm should not be used to control the arm. Assessment of subclavicular portion of pectoralis involves abduction at 90 degrees from the body. The tendon of pectoralis at the sternum should not palpate as tense even at maximum abduction of the arm.

Assessment of Shortened Trapezius (Upper)
20. The sitting patient's neck is side flexed without flexion, extension or rotation, while the opposite shoulder is stabilized from above. The range is compared on each side and palpation discovers location of shortened fibres. If sitting is not possible then, in a supine position, the same procedure is carried out with the ear being approximated to the shoulder.

Assessment of Shortened Levator Scapulae
21. Patient supine lying with arms alongside the body. The arm on the side to be tested is flexed above the head, and abducted towards the head, elbow flexed to approximately 90 degrees, so that the palm of that hand is facing ceiling ward and lies behind the patient's neck/upper back. The operator steadies the head with one hand, and steadies the shoulder on the side being assessed with the other by caudad pressure on the elevated and abducted elbow.

   Maximum flexion of the cervical spine is introduced, together with rotation and side-bending away from the side being assessed. If the levator scapulae is shortened then the range of movement is decreased and the insertion on the scapulae is painful on palpation. Shortness of this muscle often results in pain on the spinous process of C2 and the upper border of the scapula.

The examples given are not definitive, for there are many other methods of assessment of short postural muscles. Ideal methods for treating these are muscle energy procedures in which the physiological responses of post-isometric relaxation and or reciprocal inhibition are used to achieve painless stretching of shortened tissues. The key to success is identification of shortened fibres and introduction of painless muscle energy procedures (employing far less than full strength during resisted contractions and care with subsequent passive stretching). This will ensure the release of the shortening and tightness which prevents normal function.

Exercise 13.
Spend some time comparing the results of muscle tests as described above with the finding you made when searching for trigger points and other reflex activity. Are muscles which house such points always short on testing? Usually or only sometimes? Begin the final exercises in this chapter with you and your partner running through all the assessments of postural muscles, noting on a chart those which are found to be shortened. Results should then be compared with

findings obtained after practising basic spinal NMT (or abdominal NMT) assessment, in which a note is kept on a chart of all areas, points, zones of soft tissue dysfunction (palpating as abnormal, indurated, contracted as well as sensitive). Also practise Nimmo's assessment sequence.

Professor Philip Greenman D.O., in his book *Principles of Manual Medicine* describes a pattern of palpation of muscle in the spinal region which is well worth carrying out, many times, until the tissues he asks you to feel for are indeed clearly noted. The following is a summary of part of his 'palpation prescription' for this region, which commences with superfical palpation, always an exercise worth repeating.

Exercise 14.

a. Sit or stand facing the patient's back and place your hands and fingers onto the upper portion of their scapulae, just overlaying the spines of these bones. Palpate the skin for variations in temperature, tone, texture, thickness and elasticity, as you move your hands downwards over the shoulder blades.

b. At the starting position move the hands slowly and sequentially in all directions so that the skin moves on the subcutaneous fascia, and assess the degree of adherence between skin and fascia.

c. Gently lift skin between thumb and index finger and perform skin rolling, moving medially and then laterally as well as superiorly, from whichever point you started palpating. This elicits information as to the thickness and pliability of the skin as well as giving information about painful tissues. Do this on both sides of the spine, symmetrically, and compare findings.

Exercise 15.

a. Move the hands to more central point and place the fingers of one hand so that they straddle the spine, one or two fingers on each side, close to the spine, between the shoulder blades. Palpate the skin, moving it in various directions to assess the skin adherence. Compare the findings with those you assessed in tissue more lateral to the spine.

b. Now palpate through the skin in this region to the subcutaneous fascia, right down to the ligamentous structure (supraspinous) which lies between the segments, in the interspinous space. Compare its feel to the way it feels as it inserts into the spinous process. Palpate the spinous process and note the feel of bone, overlayed by skin and ligament.

b. Resting a finger on each of two or three interspaces, at this level, have the patient slowly bend their head forwards and backwards on each other. Spend some time doing this, gaining a sense of 'end-feel' of the ranges of motion involved.

Exercise 16.

a. Now place the fingers of one hand on the soft tissues between the spine and the scapula on that side. Feel through the skin and subcutaneous fascia until you are aware of the fascia which overlays the first layer of muscle. Identify the direction in which the fibres of this muscle layer travel. Have the patient draw their shoulder blade towards the spine as you continue to palpate. This movement should highlight the horizontal fibres of the trapezius muscle which you are palpating.

b. Move your pressure deeper to the next layer of muscle on one side, the rhomboid, and try to feel for the oblique direction of its pull, from above downwards. As you palpate this with one hand you can highlight the action of these fibres by having the patient draw their bent elbow (on the same side) downwards against counter-pressure offered by your free hand.

c. Going yet deeper, feel for a muscle which has a more fibrous, ropy, texture which runs vertically alongside the spine. Movement of your contact from side to side will help identify these fibres, which probably belong to the longissimus muscle, part of the erector spinae group.

d. Move your palpating contact to the side of this ropy bundle, closer to the spine, and go more deeply in order to find evidence of a deeper layer of muscles – the rotatores and multifidi – which run from one segment to another providing fine control movement possibilities. Their direction of pull is obliquely from the spine outwards (as in the case of the rhomboids in b.).

Dr Greenman suggests that you try to identify any of the small muscles which are tender, more 'full and tense', and which are therefore involved in a degree of local dysfunction.

e. Moving to the outside of the longissimus muscle (c) palpate deeply into the fascial tissue; with the angle of your palpation being somewhat towards the spine, introduce a movement upwards and downwards, as you feel for the hollows and rises of the transverse processes and the interspaces between them.

In this chapter on muscle palpation you have been exposed to a variety of approaches useful for uncovering evidence awaiting discovery. Now add this to the knowledge gained in the previous chapter.

Exercise 17. Compare your findings regarding trigger points and other palpable changes (such as neurolymphatic reflex points) as outlined in this chapter with the methods of assessment described in the previous chapter. Can you combine skin assessment with any of the methods of Lief, Nimmo, Chapman or Beal?

In the next section the methods used are no longer looking for structural change alone, but are concerned with the altered function which accompanies altered structure. Some of the methods are subtle, others less so. All are of proven value if the practitioner has the patience to develop the acuteness of touch needed for their application.

Source of Pain: Is it Reflex or Local?

Palpation of an area which the patient reports to be painful will produce increased sensitivity or tenderness if the pain is originating from that area. If, however, palpation produces no such increase in sensitivity, then the chances are strong that the pain is being referred from elsewhere. But where is it coming from?

Knowledge of the patterns of probable targets of distribution of trigger point symptoms can allow for a swift focusing on suitable sites in which to search for an offending trigger (if the pain is coming from a myofascial trigger). The discomfort could, however, be a radicular symptom coming from the spine. When pain is being referred into a limb due to a spinal problem, the greater the pain distally from the source, the greater 'the index of difficulty (the further distal, the more difficult) in applying quickly successful treatment', reports Gregory Grieve F.C.S.P. (*Mobilisation of the Spine*).

Dvorak and Dvorak (*Manual Medicine : Diagnostics*) state:

> For patients with acute radicular syndrome there is little diagnostic difficulty, which is not the case for patients with chronic back pain, some differentiation for further therapy is especially important, although not always simple.

Noting that a mixed clinical picture is common, they then say,

> When testing for the radicular syndrome, particular attention is to be paid to the motor disturbances and the deep tendon reflexes. When examining sensory radicular disorders, the attention should be towards the algesias.

However, the referred pain may not be from either a trigger or the spine. Kellgren (*Clinical Science*, 3: 175, 1938 and 4: 35, 1939) showed that:

> The superficial fascia of the back, the spinous processes and the supraspinous ligaments induce local pain upon stimulation, while stimulation of the superficial portions of the interspinous ligaments and the superficial muscles results in a diffused (more widespread) type of pain.

Clearly ligaments and fascia must be considered as sources of referred pain, and this is made clearer by Brugger ('Pseudoradikulare Syndrome', *Acta Rheumatol* 18: 1, 1960) who describes a number of syndromes in which altered arthromuscular components produce reflexogenic pain. These are attributed to painfully stimulated tissues (origins of tendons, joint capsules, and so on) producing pain in muscles, tendons and overlaying skin.

As an example, irritation and increased sensitivity in the region of the sternum, clavicles and rib attachments to the sternum, through occupational or postural patterns, will influence or cause painful intercostal muscles, scalenes, sternomastoid, pectoralis major and cervical muscles. The increased tone in these muscles and the resultant stresses which they produce may lead to spondylogenic problems in the cervical region, with further spread of symptoms. Overall this syndrome can produce chronic pain in the neck, head, chest wall, arm and hand (even mimicking heart disease).

Dvorak and Dvorak have charted a multitude of what they term 'spondylogenic reflexes' which derive from (in the main) intervertebral joints. The palpated changes are characterized as:

> Painful swellings, tender upon pressure and detachable with palpation, located in the musculofascial tissue in topographically well defined sites. The average size varies from 0.5 cm to 1 cm and the main characteristic is the absolutely timed and qualitative linkage to the extent of the functionally abnormal position (segmental dysfunction). As long as a disturbance exists, the zones of irritation can be identified, yet disappear immediately after the removal of the disturbance.

Dvorak and Dvorak see altered mechanics in a vertebral unit as causing 'reflexogenic pathological change of the soft tissue, the most important being the "myotendinoses", which can be identified by palpation'. Some would argue that the soft tissue changes precede the altered vertebral states, at least in some instances (poor posture, overuse, misuse, abuse). Wherever you stand in this debate, this brief survey of some opinions as to 'where the pain is coming from', shows clearly that we need to keep many possibilities in mind.

Chapter 5

Palpation of Muscle Function
(Including Circulation of CSF and 'Energy'; and 'Has Tissue a Memory?')

The functional aspects of soft tissue palpation contained in this chapter do not include assessments of muscle strength/weakness, not because this is unimportant, but because there are texts in abundance which cover this ground more than adequately already. Vladimir Janda's *Muscle Function Testing* is recommended.

Once again we can turn to Viola Frymann for an introduction to this complex subject of palpation of muscle function, as she describes what we should expect as we begin to palpate muscular tissues for anything other than their mechanical status:

> If the hand is laid on a healthy muscle mass, of a resting limb, it is possible in the space of a few seconds to 'tune in' to the inherent motion within. A state of rapport, of fluid continuity between the examiner, and the examined is established and a whole new realm of exploration lies ahead. The continuity of fluid within the body is never interrupted in health – intra and inter-cellular fluid, lymph, cerebrospinal fluid – and it is in a constant state of rhythmic, fluctuant motion.

Frymann maintains that the vitality of tissue can be judged by the strength of such motions, with a wide variety of grades of tissue vitality being apparent. The example is given of the difference in the 'feel' noted when a previously paralysed and a presently paralysed limb are palpated. In the first a mere 'murmur' of motion will be felt, whereas in the latter there will be no detectable rhythmic motion at all. Frymann goes further and states that judgement can also be made as to the likelihood of improvement, based on information such as this.

Exercise 1. If you have access to someone with a totally or partially paralysed limb (stroke victim?) Frymann suggests you start by simultaneously placing one hand on the spinal segment which supplies the principle innervation to the affected limb, and the other on the affected limb.

Having done this pause for a few minutes, all the while concentrating on any 'activity' under your hands. The spinal hand should begin to register the rhythm. The degree to which the ('rhythmic integrated') response is subsequently felt in the other hand is the key to potential viability of the presently paralysed tissue. Frymann calls this communication – which in normal tissue has a surging, rhythmic, nature – 'the vital fluid tide' within.

What is the rhythmic 'fluid tide' which can be felt when we palpate? As in our investigation of the skin (see Chapter 3) it is necessary to come to an understanding of aspects of physiological function as it relates to this 'vital fluid tide', most notably how cerebrospinal fluid circulates, possibly throughout the whole body, as well as something of the trophic function of nerves.

Ehrlinghauser's Research   For a deeper understanding of the concepts being discussed here, the reader is referred to the article 'The Circulation of CSF through the connective tissue system' by Ralph Ehrlinghauser D.O. in the *Academy of Applied Osteopathy Yearbook 1959* as well as to the book *Craniosacral Therapy* by Upledger and Vredevoogd.

Ehrlinghauser starts his discussion with the news that research has demonstrated that collagen (connective tissue) has a tubular structure (Kennedy J., Tubular structure of collagen fibrils. *Science* 121: 673–4, May 6 1955 and Wyckoff R., Fine Structure of Connective Tissues in Foundation Conferences on Connective Tissues No. 3 1952 p.p.38–91) a discovery which, he believes, will revolutionize our understanding of human physiology. Cerebro Spinal Fluid (CSF) motion is considered by cranial osteopaths to play a major part in controlling a vital 'semi-closed' hydraulic system. This is bounded by the cranial vaults themselves and the dural membranes which, together, form the semi-closed aspects of the unit.

CSF enters and leaves this hydraulic system via the choroid plexuses and the arachnoid villae. As well as giving shape and stability (and, some believe, motion) to this system, the largely incompressible CSF also fluctuates through the tubular collagen fibrils of the connective tissues throughout the body, CSF is seen to act as a transport medium between the subarachnoid space and cells of the body.

The discovery of collagen's tubular structure indicates that, far from connective tissue being merely structurally supportive (as it anatomically connects epithelial, muscular and nervous tissues) it can also be assumed to be linked to these tissues histologically, biochemically, physiologically and of course pathologically, when dysfunction/disease is present. Connective tissue, with its hollow, tubular fibril structure, is continuous throughout the body, from the fascia of the skull to that of the feet. It provides fascial planes, envelopes, reflections and spaces, as well as ligaments and tendons, giving protection, cohesion, form, shape and support to the circulatory, lymphatic and nervous systems which it separates, shapes and binds.

In 1939, W.G. Sutherland D.O., having established that the cranial bones had a constant rhythmic physiological range of motion, postulated that CSF fluctuation provided the mechanism which moved these. Subsequent studies have confirmed that, although sutures provide a strong bond between cranial bones, they do allow movement. Other workers have considered that such motion as is observed relates to variations in venous, arterial and respiratory pressures, and these do undoubtedly influence matters.

It is also considered that there exist, within the brain, cells which provide a further rhythmic pulsation which influences fluid motion (the oligodendroglia). Pulsations of between 6 and 12 per minute are now established as the norm in good health for what has been termed the primary respiratory mechanism in cranial oesteopathy. These rhythms are unrelated to normal respiration or heart rate, and are seen to operate in all mammals. Research indicates that oxygen reaches fine neural structures at this rate (8 to 12 waves per minute) and that administration of carbon dioxide (30 per cent) stops the waves in humans. In animal studies administration to anaesthetized dogs of concentrations of carbon dioxide leads to a precipitous rise in CSF pressure.

In the rhythmical coiling and uncoiling of the oligodendroglial cells, which provide at least part of the pulsating impetus for CSF fluctuation, we therefore have one explanation for its motive power through the channels which exist within connective tissue. Erlinghauser provides ample research validation for this concept (much simplified in this account) of the circulation of CSF, from the subarachnoid spaces via tubular collagen fibrils to the intercellular spaces, where it combines with tissue fluids, being in turn reabsorbed by the end-lymph vessels, into the lymph system and thence to the venous system. This leads naturally enough to the conclusion that any derangement of the connective tissue system must result in limitations to the physiological flow of CSF within the collagen fibrils, with negative consequences to cellular health.

If we want to obtain palpatory evidence of dysfunction affecting the musculoskeletal system (which will always involve connective tissue) the ability of the palpator to 'read' the rhythmic pulsation of CSF becomes very important indeed. This is the 'vital fluid' which Frymann referred to in the opening paragraphs of this chapter.

Upledger places a different emphasis on factors involved in the motive force which drives the fluid fluctuations of CSF. He sees the fluid structure of this system as being 'primarily biphasic', with more or less stationary viscous fluid at the inner core and a lighter almost non-viscous CSF externally. The hydraulic contents of the system are, says Upledger:

> Subjected to the pulsatory motions of the arterial system, the venous system and the pulmonary system which transmits its effect to the dura mater through the vertebral connections along the cervical section of the spinal column. The lateral displacements which all these systems induce upon the fluid region set the latter into motion.

Whether the Erlinghauser or the Upledger model is more accurate is largely a side issue. What matters in our palpation studies is the fact that fluid fluctuations occur, that they can be palpated and they have significance. Upledger summarizes the cranial (and other osseous and soft tissue) motions which result from or take part in the rhythmic motion of CSF. Recall that this has a rhythm of 6 to 12 cycles per minute under normal circumstances. Primary respiratory flexion is the term applied to the extreme range of motion occurring during each of these cycles, at which time the head becomes wider transversely and shorter in its antero-posterior dimension. At the same time the *entire body* externally rotates and widens. There is then a brief pause before the body returns to the starting position, termed extension, during which time the head narrows and elongates as the rest of the body goes into internal rotation. All these motions are very slight indeed but once you learn of their existence palpation of them during the approximately 6 seconds of a full cycle, can be learned fairly quickly. Upledger says, 'Once you tune into these motions, you can perceive your own body doing flexion-extension cycles as you stand or walk. After a time you will learn to tune yourself in and out of your own physiological body motion as well.'

One other anatomical link needs to be explained regarding this concept; the cranial link to the sacrum. The connection between the occiput and the sacrum is the dural membrane, which is itself continuous with the meningeal membranes. If the occiput moves forward as the flexion phase of cranial respiratory cycle commences, it will create a synchronous movement (pull) of the sacral base, which moves posteriorly during this phase (taking the sacral apex and coccyx anteriorly).

What should we be trying to learn from our palpation of these rhythms and cycles? Upledger summarizes:

From the diagnostic, prognostic and therapeutic points of view, we are interested in a qualitative estimate of the strength of the inherent energy which is driving the physiological motion, the symmetry of the body motion response (both of the craniosacral system and of the extrinsic body

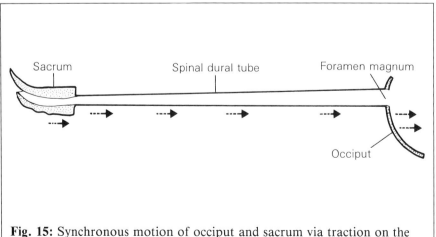

Fig. 15: Synchronous motion of occiput and sacrum via traction on the dural tube.

connective tissues), and in the range and quality of each cyclical motion. Is it fighting against a resistance barrier?

Not only is there useful information available when palpating the cranial and sacral components of this complex, but it is possible to feel the cycle in any tissues of the body, even in patients who are in a vegetative state.

Exercise 2. Go back to Chapter 2 and do again exercise 17, 19 and 20 which focused attention on cranial and sacral rhythms. Follow these with the following exercise.

Your partner/patient lies on his/her side, pillow under the head in order to avoid any side-bending of the neck. You are seated behind and place one hand on the occiput (fingers going over the crown) and the other on the sacrum, fingers towards the coccyx.

Palpate the motions of the occiput and the sacrum. Are they synchronous? When you have satisfied yourself (five minutes should be ample) have the model remove the pillow, so that the neck is side-bent.

Repalpate and compare the results. Are the rhythmic pulsations still synchronous?

Exercise 3. With your partner/patient prone or seated palpate the paraspinal musculature for craniosacral motion. Upledger suggests

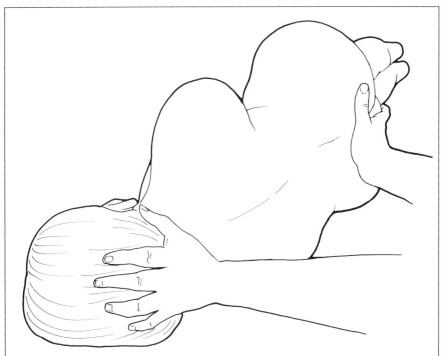

Fig. 16: Examination for synchrony of motion between occiput and sacrum.

this be done so that the spinous processes lie between your fingers. When a muscle has been denervated, he says, the rhythm will rise to 20 to 30 cycles per minute, which can help to differentiate pain from nerve root compression from other sources of pain.

Upledger again emphasizes that practice is the only way to gain confidence in this form of palpation. 'Do not let your intellect obstruct the development of your palpatory skills.' He is of course right to repeat this, for initially the 'feeling' of motion is nothing more than that, and is easily discounted by the mind.

Note: I suggest that in all early exercises in which cranial motion or craniosacral rhythms are being assessed the student of palpation should think in terms of a slight 'surging' sensation, sometimes described as feeling 'as though the tide is coming in', or a feeling of 'fullness' under the palpating hand, rather than expecting to feel movement of a grosser form. After a few seconds this 'surge' will be felt to recede, the tide goes out again. This is a subtle sensation, but once you have tuned into it, it is unmistakable, and very real indeed.

Exercise 4. Have your partner/patient lie face upwards. You stand at the foot of the couch cradling one foot (heel) in each hand. Close your eyes and feel for external rotation of the leg during the flexion phase of the craniosacral cycle and internal rotation as it returns to neutral during the extension phase.

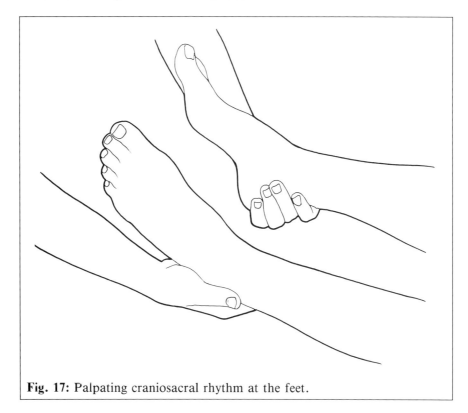

Fig. 17: Palpating craniosacral rhythm at the feet.

Once you have become acutely aware of this motion compare the ease of motion in the rotation of the two legs.

Does there seem to be an easier feel to the external or the internal rotation, symmetrically in one or other of the legs?

Upledger's books are a treasure house of information for anyone who wishes to add craniosacral work to their repertoire. Instruction in workshop or seminar settings is, however, essential before this is applied therapeutically.

It is both possible and desirable during palpatory training for the student to learn to stop the cranial cycles, a process known as inducing the 'still' point. This can be done from many places in the body, for example from the feet as in Exercise 4, or from the sacrum or occiput.

What is required is that the palpating hands follow the palpated part as it goes to the limit of the flexion or extension phase, and to lock the part(s) there, not applying pressure, simply restraining the tendency to go into the next phase of the cycle. This is repeated after subsequent cycles until the rhythm stops completely, for some seconds or even minutes. This is the 'still' point (see Exercise 5).

After a while the palpating (restraining) hand(s) will again feel the movement try to start. This is then allowed and a general improvement is usually seen in the amplitude and symmetry of the motion. Therapeutically this has the effect of enhancing fluid motion, restoring flexibility and reducing congestion.

Exercise 5. As an exercise in establishing a 'still' point go back to Exercise 4 and, when you have established a clear rhythm of external and internal rotation of the legs during the flexion and extension phases of the craniosacral fluid fluctuation, start to follow the external rotation while preventing any return to internal rotation of the legs when this phase is perceived. Do not forcibly rotate the legs, simply go with the external rotation each time it occurs, taking up additional slack to its limit, and then prevent any return to the neutral position. After a number of pulsations (Upledger says anywhere from 5 to 20 repetitions), during which a slight increased external rotation will be achieved, the impulses will cease.

There may be sensations of tremor, shuddering or pulling noted through the contact hands from elsewhere in the system (as the cranial impulses try to deal with the restriction) but eventually this will cease and the 'still' point will have been reached. During this phase the patient will relax deeply, breathing may alter and corrections occur spontaneously within the musculoskeletal system.

Note: The 'still' point may easily be initiated via cranial and sacral structures but practising of this approach on such structures is not recommended without guidance, as it is all too easy to traumatize the delicate craniosacral mechanisms.

From a palpation point of view this is as far as we can go with cranial fluid fluctuations. Just how this is integrated into an individual's practice must hinge on the degree of interest this avenue excites, and how much cranial study is undertaken.

Energy Upledger's writings and research also take us into another dimension of 'flow' through the tissues we are palpating: energy. This is clearly an area which many find difficult to deal with, either intellectually or practically. The best advice the author can give is that you suspend disbelief, attempt the various exercises which are outlined below – based on the work of Becker, Smith and Upledger, amongst others – and see what you feel. Whether or not you accept the explanations which these respected researchers and clinicians give for 'their' approach to reading and manipulating what that conceive as energy fluctuations in the body is quite another matter.

If you have patience, you will undoubtedly feel movements and rhythms as you follow the exercises given below, and for the purpose of learning to 'feel' you are asked to accept that these represent, in one form or another, 'energy'. In Chapter 8 we will be looking at even more subtle energy manifestations, as used in methods such as Therapeutic Touch and the discussion below should be kept in mind as that chapter is studied, for we are entering an area which is ill-defined, where function and concepts of energy interactions are mixed and blurred.

That something palpable exists which is called energy by numerous researchers and practitioners is not in question. What remains controversial is its nature and function. Dr Smith outlines his model of energy patterns within and around the body. There is a non-differentiated field which pervades the body, which extends some distance beyond the limits of the physical body. Currents which move within us are organized into:

1. a deep layer which flows through the skeletal system;
2. a middle layer which flows through the soft tissues (neurovascular bundles, fascia, muscle cleavages, and so on) as described in Traditional Chinese Medicine, and;
3. a superficial layer which is found just below the skin.

These energy patterns are capable of disruption if the physical medium through which they pass (bone, soft tissue, skin) is traumatized or stressed, and the non-differentiated field may carry 'imprints' of imbalances caused by physical, toxic or emotional insults and traumas, especially if these have not been absorbed by specific tissues or systems. Before examining the work of Fritz Smith M.D. and Rollin Becker D.O., in relation to such energy patterns, we should become familiar with Upledger's concept of the 'energy cyst'.

One of the palpable phenomena of the energy system is said to be the chakras, or energy centres, which are situated as specific sites on the body, and which can be palpated on the surface or just off the surface. The original concept of chakras was Ayurvedic (Indian) as was the word prahna (energy) used to describe the vital 'substance' with which they are associated. The palpable energy centres are characterized by the clockwise circulation of energy at these places. They are said to range in size from about 3 to 15 centimetres in diameter and number 7 in all:

- The root chakra is palpated just above the pubis, Upledger suggests, with one hand under the sacrum and the other resting on the lower abdomen. It relates to sexual function.
- The navel chakra is best palpated similarly, one hand under the lumbar spine, the other just below the navel (no hand pressure, just a touch). This relates to emotions and sensitivity.
- The spleen chakra is best palpated, says Upledger, with one hand over the lumbodorsal junction and the other over the epigastrium. It relates to energy assimilation and immunity.
- The heart chakra requires one hand under the mid-thoracic spine and the other touching the central sternal area. It relates to emotions connected with love and 'hurt' feelings.
- The throat chakra should be palpated with one hand behind the neck and the other over the centre of the throat. It may be felt as two centres of spinning energy. It relates to personal communication and relationships.
- The brow chakra may be palpated with a hand under the occiput and three fingers over the glabella. It has an intense energy 'feel' relating as it does to intuitive perception.
- The crown chakra is palpated at the crown of the head where it may be felt as an energy outflow rather than a spinning energy centre, related, it is said, to the pineal gland and to spiritual factors.

It is not necessary to accept the existence of chakras as such in order to palpate them, they can be seen merely as places where circulating energy is more organized or dense.

Exercise 6. Palpate the chakras as outlined above. Do you sense any surge, vibration, churning, fluctuation of motion?

This is an exercise to come back to, after completing some of the work suggested in further exercises below, if the chakra concept interests you.

Both Traditional Chinese Medicine and Ayurvedic medicine hold that there are channels over the surface of the body, and within it, which are conduits for the flow of energy. If these are blocked or altered the result is dysfunction or disease. There are abundant texts which help the interested reader to a greater awareness of both chakras and the meridian system.

Restricted Energy Flow: The Varma and Upledger Models

It may be useful to consider a similarity in the ideas of two different researchers, separated by time and culture, whose concepts were very close, if not identical. Stanley Lief D.C., the developer of neuromuscular technique was greatly influenced by Dr Dewanchand Varma, an Ayurvedic practitioner working in Paris in the early 1930s, whose method of treatment of energy imbalances utilized a primitive form of NMT which he called 'pranotherapy'.

In his book *The Human Machine and its Forces* Varma discussed the ways in which 'electro-magnetic currents' derived from the atmosphere (at the chakras) were capable of becoming obstructed, 'by certain adhesions in which the muscular fibres harden together so that the nervous currents can no longer pass through them'. It was his method of pranotherapy, a sort of manual soft tissue manipulation, which would release these palpable obstructions, and which Lief incorporated into NMT.

Varma mentions changes in the skin when such obstructions occur, saying 'If the skin becomes attached to the underlying muscle, the current cannot pass, the part loses its sensibility.' This is remarkably close to Dr Lewit's description of hyperalgesic skin zones is it not?

How were the obstructions and adhesions dealt with? Varma suggested a two-stage 'treatment', which – as in NMT, is actually an assessment – during which treatment is imparted, or not, as the therapist deems appropriate. The first part of the assessment/treatment involved the tissues being prepared by 'rubbing with oil'. The actual 'manipulation' of the tissues was performed by first 'separating' skin from underlying tissue, followed by a gentle 'separation' of the muscle fibres, a process which required 'highly sensitive fingers able to distinguish between thick and thin fibres, and...highly developed consciousness and sensitivity, attained by hours of patient daily practice on the living body'.

While these are descriptions of some interest they fail to instruct adequately; what did Varma actually do? My uncle Boris Chaitow D.C. (who at the time of writing is still in practice, in his early 80s) was co-developer of NMT (with his cousin Stanley Lief). Chaitow has commented on Varma's methods (personal communication); the most valuable essential which he derived from Varma came as a result of having treatment from him. It was during one of these sessions that the 'variable pressure' factor become apparent, something which Chaitow still holds to be invaluable in both assessment and treatment. This subtle factor, which allows the palpating hand/digit to 'meet the tissues', not overwhelm them, is a factor which will be seen again when we come to examine the research work of Fritz Smith M.D. (see p.115 below).

Dr John Upledger (*Craniosacral Therapy 11: Beyond the Dura*) describes how his concept of an 'energy cyst' developed as he worked with biophysicists, psychologists, biochemists, neurophysiologists and others at the Michigan State University College of Osteopathic Medicine:

> The energy cyst is a construct of our imagination which may have objective reality. We believe that it manifests as an obstruction to the efficient conduction of electricity through the body tissues (primarily fasciae) where it resides, acts as an irritant contributing to the development of the facilitated segment [see Chapter 4] and as a localized irritable focus.

Varma hypothesized his 'obstructions' to energy flow over fifty years before Upledger's development of the 'energy cyst' theory, which is quite remarkably similar.

(There is no suggestion whatever that Upledger or his fellow workers had, or have, any knowledge of Varma and his work, which quite simply vanished almost without trace during the Second World War.)

Upledger believes that the cyst interrupts the flow of *chi*, the Chinese term for energy, and that by palpation these obstructions can be readily found. They can result, says Upledger, from trauma, infection, physiological dysfunction (see commentary in Chapter 4 as to how soft tissue changes occur and progress) mental or emotional problems, or through disturbance of the chakras.

What do 'energy cysts' feel like? 'The cyst is hotter, more energetic, less organised and less functional than surrounding tissues.'

How does Upledger pinpoint a 'cyst'? He uses a method which he terms interference arcing, in which he 'feels' for waves, or arcs of energy, relating to such dysfunctional centres. The cysts seem to generate interference waves which can be sensed (usually pulsating at a much faster rate than normal tissue) superimposed on the normal rhythms of tissue.

If these waves can be imagined as being like ripples on a pond surface after a pebble has disturbed the surface, it is possible to visualize that the palpating hands could 'zero in' on the centre of the wave pattern, to locate the source, the 'cyst'.

It would not matter from which direction, in relation to the 'cyst', the hands were coming in their palpation, for the centre would remain constant, as would the wave pattern.

(Compare the image of an 'energy cyst' as pictured by Upledger with that of the 'eye' of the disturbance which Becker describes in his work on p.126. For more details of Upledger's palpation see p.131.)

Exercise 7. Palpate the soft tissues of your patient/partner, in an area of dysfunction, trigger points or other reflex activity previously identified, using the methods of Lewit, Lief or Nimmo, for cysts/arcs, as described above. Can you sense the waves?

Fritz Smith M.D. has explained his concepts and methods in his book *Inner Bridges*. He has called his approach 'zero balancing', but it is the book's sub-title *A guide to energy movement and body structure* which gives the strongest clue as to the way he thinks and the imbalances and changes he is looking for, and hoping to correct, in therapy.

He describes the following realization, after ten years of study of both orthodox and traditional (mainly Oriental) medical methods:

During this process I came to recognise a specific area in a person where movement and structure are in juxtaposition, similar to the situation in a sailboat where the wind (movement) and the sail (structure) meet. From the explanation of the interface, in 1973, I formulated the structural acupressure system of Zero Balancing, to evaluate and balance the relationship between energy and structure.

His book is not an instruction manual, but rather examines the relationship between ancient energy concepts and modern medicine, Eastern esoteric anatomy and Western human anatomy, subjective inner experiences and objective observation. This approach is of considerable value and importance to those practitioners who struggle to align the apparent contradictions faced when comparing the variables in theory and methodology which exist between Western and Eastern medicine.

Smith examines what he terms 'the foundations for the energetic bridge' and looks at, among other areas, 'foundation joints'. These, he says, are the cranial bones of the skull, the sacroiliac articulations, the intercarpal articulations of the hand, the pubic symphysis and the intertarsal articulations of the foot. These, he maintains, transmit and balance the energetic forces of the body, rather than being merely involved in movement and locomotion. What they have in common is that they have small ranges of motion and little or no voluntary movement potential. In all cases movement in them occurs in response to forces acting upon the area, rather than being initiated by the part itself.

Thus, if there is an imbalance or altered function in any of these joints, the body is obliged to compensate for the problem rather than being able to resolve the situation through adaptation. Such compensation can be widespread and will often involve other associated structures, commonly becoming 'locked into' the body, limiting its ability to function.

Smith believes that these joints have the closest relationship with the subtle body and any limitation in them, he suggests, can be seen as a direct read-out of the energetic component of the body. He reminds us of the basic law of physics which tells us that *the effect of stress on any mechanism will spread until it is absorbed or until the mechanism breaks down.*

What Smith is pointing to is the fact that stresses will spread into these 'foundation areas' and that, because they have no power of voluntary motion, they will absorb the strains until these become locked into them, or until there is a resolution of normality by outside forces. Clearly from a vantage point which looks at the effects of joint dysfunction on muscles inserting into such structures, we can see that there is the likelihood of continued stress, leading to their shortening and contraction (see Chapter 4).

If we think of the ramifications of pelvic dysfunction on the local musculature (piriformis, quadratus, psoas, and so on) and the possibility that changes in these soft tissues can produce pelvic (including SI and pubic) stresses, we can see the advantages of being able to identify and release such contractions, as discussed in Chapter 4.

Smith also identifies other 'semi-foundation' joints, such as the intervertebral articulations, rib joints (costovertebral, costochondral, costotransversus) and the clavicular articulations with the first rib and sternum. He uses a variety of assessment methods in order to identify reduction in normal energy flow in associated tissues, and describes methods which he uses to restore this function when reduced energy flow is perceived. He makes much of the usefulness in assessment of the ability to identify end of motion range in joint play (discussed in the notes on page 151).

Smith's work, therefore, seems to be a bridge between the gross methods of Western physiological methodology and the apparently abstract concepts of 'energy' medicine. He explains the way he makes contact with the patient. He calls this 'essential touch' saying, quite rightly, that it is common in bodywork to be touched only on the physical level, not to have a significant energetic interchange take place. The connection which he wants to achieve transcends the physical touching and involves an instinctive, intuitive, yet conscious action on the part of the aware therapist.

What should we feel when this is achieved? Dr Smith describes it thus:

> There are a number of sensations, mostly involving the feeling of movement or aliveness, which let us know we are engaging an energy field. We may perceive a fine vibration in the other person's body or in the aura, a feeling we are making contact with a low voltage current. This may be described as tingling, buzzing, a chill sensation, 'goose bumps', as well as a subtle sensation that some people describe as 'vibration'. We may also perceive a grosser feeling of movement as though the person's body, or our own, were expanding or contracting, even though we see no physical change.

This is not dissimilar to Frymann's description early in this chapter. Smith uses the concept of a fulcrum in order to establish his contact, as do other workers in this field notably, Becker and Lief, although in each case the descriptions of their individual 'fulcrums' are quite different. A fulcrum is defined, says Smith, as a balance point, a position, element or agency through, around, or by means of which vital powers are exercised:

> The simplest fulcrum is created by the direct pressure of one or more fingers into the body, to form a firm support, around which the body can orient.

The fulcrum needs to be 'deep' enough into the body so that the physical slack of the tissue is taken up; this is the point at which any further pressure meets with resistance in the tissue beneath the fingers. *Getting 'in touch' with the person's energy field is thus achieved by taking up slack from tissues, so that any additional movement on our part will be translated directly into the person's experience.*

Compare this description with the request, by Lief and Chaitow, that digital or hand pressure in NMT be 'variable', matching that of the tissues it is meeting.

Exercise 8. Smith suggests we learn to practise this approach using a water-filled balloon, 10 inches or so in diameter. Place this on a table and slip your fingers under it, raise them and be sensitive to the pressure on your finger tips. As the fingers are raised, slack is taken out of your own tissues as well as the slack of the balloon. As you increase pressure there comes a moment when you 'connect' with the mass of water in the balloon and at that moment the finger tips are acting as a fulcrum for the balloon:

> At any fulcrum or balance point one is in solid contact with the material, the mass orients around the finger, and any further pressure will affect the energy.

Note: Smith insists that there should be frequent breaks (he calls these 'disconnects') from the patient when energy exercises (or therapy) are being performed. A loss of sensitivity – which he calls 'accommodation' – takes place as well as a draining of the therapist's vital reserves.

Other ways of creating a fulcrum, apart from direct pressure with finger or hand, can involve stretching, twisting, bending or sliding contacts.

> **Exercise 9.** Smith suggests you take a rubber band and stretch it, taking out the slack. At that point he likens what you have done to 'making contact' in the patient situation. Any further movement or stretch will involve the rubber itself. With this, and the balloon, in mind, contact with your patient by placing a hand onto their tissues, anywhere, and lightly pull the hand towards yourself and slightly 'lift' it from the tissues.
>
> Smith describes this as a 'half-moon' vector, since it combines both lifting and pulling motions which translate into a curved pull. This is the key to what he seeks.
>
> Once you have taken out the physical slack, and have established an interface (fulcrum) with the tissues *any additional movement on your part will be felt by the patient and any movement in the person's body will be felt by you.*
>
> At this point you are in touch at the energy level.
>
> Can you feel it?
>
> Stay with the contact for some time and assess what you feel.

It is with such a contact, Smith states, that you should feel vibrations and currents, and by adding more movement yourself you can judge how the tissue (or the patient as a whole) responds. To fine-tune the fulcrum contact he asks himself 'How does this feel to the patient?' or 'How would this feel if it were done to me?'

The response helps him decide whether to pull harder or more gently, to twist more, or less. He also asks the patient how it feels to them, suggesting that with a straight pressure fulcrum a 'nice hurt' is what is desirable.

Long before I was aware of Dr Smith's work (but possibly after reading of Dr Becker's ideas) I came to use a contact which achieves similar results in a diagnostic sense to that described by Dr Smith. I make a hand, mainly a palm, contact, with fingers lightly touching, but not usually involved. I try to think of the palm as though I were

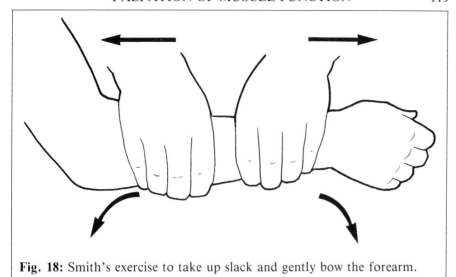

Fig. 18: Smith's exercise to take up slack and gently bow the forearm.

applying a suction pad to glass. Lifting and slightly turning the cupped contact until there is a feel of 'suction' between my hand and the patient. The writhing, pulsating or flickering sensations of the energy field are felt almost immediately. Try this, and see what you feel. Compare it to the 'half-moon vector' exercise above. Is it the same?

Dr Smith suggests the following 'exercises' to help in assessment of bone status.

> **Exercise 10.** Take hold of your partner/patient's forearm, above the wrist and below the elbow, and – after taking out the slack by 'pulling' your hands apart until the point is reached where you have created a fulcrum – gently put a bend or 'bow' into the arm.
>
> After taking up the slack of the physical body and soft tissues (by pulling the hands apart, see notes on 'end-feel' page 151) the resistance of the bone itself will be encountered.
>
> Any movement from this interface position will be felt by both the patient and yourself. Make a 'bowing' motion in one direction just as far as the tissues will allow, and then gently release the tension; then make a bowing motion in the opposite direction.
>
> Try this several times, once with the eyes open, and once with the eyes closed. Repeat the exercise on the person's other forearm and compare the findings.

Smith states that if the arm is normal, not injured, it may 'bow' more easily in one direction than the other; one bow may feel obstructed, or the bow may suggest a twisting motion. It may have the feel of a steel bar or be more rubbery. Great variations exist and it is up to each of us to establish what 'normal' feels like; to become aware of what is acceptable and what needs working on.

He then suggests a similar study of the long bones of the lower leg which are probably a better testing ground for practice than the forearm, which has a natural rotational tendency anyway, and so can confuse assessment.

> **Exercise 11.** Introduce a twisting motion, as if gently wringing a sweater. Place one hand just above the ankle and the other below the knee. Take up slack in the soft tissue (pull hands apart) and gently twist in one direction (hands going in opposite directions), feeling the bony resistance.
>   Repeat in the other direction.
>   What do you feel?

> Because the bones are denser in the leg than the forearm, and because the muscles are heavier, it takes a moment longer to perceive the energy currents interacting in the twisting motion. It is an exaggeration to say that energy on this level moves with the speed of molasses, but the principle is true.

(Smith)

If this exercise is performed on several people, within a short space of time, comparisons are easier. By sharing experiences with others it is possible to validate the subtle perceptions derived from these exercises. *This is not an exercise in judging whether things are good or bad, but in becoming sensitive to motions and energies not previously registered.*

If it is possible to palpate limbs which have previously been fractured and which have healed, energy current variations become very instructive:

> Energy fields across a fracture may feel heavy and dense, have low vitality, or be disorganised and chaotic. These qualities relate to the process of reconnecting or bridging the energy fields across the damaged bone.

(Smith)

Can these findings be altered? Yes, says Smith. He takes a forearm, for example, which has an old fracture, grasping it as in Exercise 9 above. He takes out the slack by stretching apart his hands:

> Holding this, I might add a further stretching force, and then, in addition, a bowing or twisting force. I hold this configuration, being sensitive to the resilience of the bone, for a brief period, possibly 15 to 20 seconds, and then gently release.

On re-evaluation he would expect a lessening of the asymmetry of the original force fields, a greater freedom of energetic movement through the long bone. He says that he allows three such attempts in order to create the greatest degree of 'shift' at any one session.

Note: I suggest, when you are trying to introduce twisting or bowing or any other direction of motion to bony structures or soft tissues, that you do not try to produce this effect by means of force from your hands alone. Having made the initial contact and allowed time for a melding of the contours of your hands with the tissues, use your arms to take out the slack, or to introduce a direction of motion. Indeed, consider the hands in this situation to be the contact only, with the motive force coming from the shoulders and arms.

If you were trying to use a spanner, to free a tight nut say, you would not use the strength of the hands alone, but would introduce the effort through the whole arm. In a far more subtle manner the motion, or direction of effort, in this sort of exercise is best achieved by very subtle, whole arm movements rather than just the hands trying to achieve the desired objective.

Anyone who has performed work on the cranium (after suitable instruction) will know that motion in the skull can be palpated or introduced in a similar manner far more effectively – and with less chance of injury – if leverage is applied by subtle use of arm muscles to guide the hand, rather than letting hand strength act alone.

Where energy motion in soft tissues is concerned, Smith tells us that a difficulty arises, since taking out the slack in pliable tissues is far less easily accomplished making the reading of energy currents in soft tissues more difficult. He suggests that a good way to start is to make two energetic contacts with the fingers and to 'read' the current as it flows from one point to the other.

> **Exercise 12.** If one finger is placed on tissue below the elbow and a finger of the other hand is placed at wrist level a sense of connection will be felt after a short while. This may be noted as a pulsation, movement, buzzing or just a sense of 'connection'. (Compare this with Exercise 10 in Chapter 2.)

Both the time taken for this 'connection' to happen, and the strength and quality of the connection should be noted as you practise.

Smith introduces the debate as to whether the right hand receives such impulses or sends them, and states his conclusion that the operator's thoughts determine the direction of flow (Upledger concurs). Let both hands be neutral, is his advice, and allow the patient's body to organize itself around your two contact 'poles', allowing these to be organizational fulcrums rather than predetermining which direction you want flow to take place.

Smith suggests that Traditional Chinese Medicine (TCM) has long used just such energy readings, most obviously in use of pulse diagnosis, and that once you have convinced yourself that you can indeed feel energy flows, it is time to start understanding the subtle ways in which you can use this information in evaluating the state of the patient. Therapy using these energy flows is only a small step beyond that stage.

Smith states that evaluation of the superficial level of internal energy flow (known as *protective chi* in TCM) is best achieved using your hands just above the body surface, as in Therapeutic Touch (Chapter 8), as well as palpating the skin texture and temperature (Chapter 3).

Beyond the energy fields which are related to the superficial soft tissue, and bones, lies an energy field which he terms 'background' energy, on which can be 'imprinted' past trauma - chemical, emotional and psychic as well as physical. This brings us close to Becker's concepts involving tissue 'memory' which we will examine below.

There is an interesting resemblance between craniosacral stillpoint

concepts and something Smith describes in energy work. Once he has
established the fulcrum between himself and the patient a number of
sensations are possible, he declares. As he holds traction he may sense
that the patient's energy body is elongating, 'stretching' or 'flowing'
into his hands, a process which at some point will stop.

If at that time there is not a feeling of contraction as though the
energy body is returning to its previous state, but rather of a stillness, a
resting in the 'elongated' state, Smith would gradually release the
traction and rest the patient's legs on the table. The patient then remains
in a very deep relaxed state for some moments before returning to
normal (he watches eye movements, patient's colour and breathing
pattern to assess states of consciousness).

However, if – for therapeutic reasons – Smith wishes to anchor the
energy field as it tries to contract again, he can do so by maintaining
traction. This would be very similar to the idea of holding the still point
as the body tried to normalize ('organize' or 'unwind') itself around that
fulcrum, in craniosacral methodology, or functional technique in
osteopathy. If, however, he were to decide to go with the retraction,
rather than anchoring it, this would be 'like letting a stretched rubber
band slowly go back to its slack position'.

Exercise 13. Introduce traction from the ankles of the supine patient
until all slack has been removed. Sense the connection with the energy
field of the patient. Does it elongate, and eventually try to contract?
If so slowly release it, like an elastic band.

Smith also suggests that we try to distinguish between palpable energy
fields which lie beyond the surface of the body and reflect present states
of body and mind (these vibrations not being 'imprinted' on the energy
field), and those patterns of energy related to forceful trauma or
stimulus of a physical, chemical, emotional or psychic nature.

These latter imbalances exist, he says, as freestanding energy wave
forms, abnormal currents, vortices, or an excess or deficiency of energy
within the field. These imprinted changes are more likely to develop in
response to trauma of a physical nature, interacting with emotional
trauma, or when a highly aroused or depressed state existed at the time
of trauma.

This combination of stress factors interacting disrupts the subtle
body. Smith uses a metaphor of 'wrinkled clothing' to describe these
changes in the subtle energy fields around us; they may disappear on
their own, or may require help to 'iron them out'.

Assessment of such changes involves two tasks. First we need to quiet
the physical body so that we can feel the deeper energy patterns. Second
we have to 'take up the slack', a common theme in Smith's work. We
can achieve this reduction in slack by means of a traction fulcrum,
through the legs, or a compression fulcrum through the shoulders.
Describing the latter he says:

I sit at the head of the table, rest my hands firmly and comfortably over the person's shoulders, and gently press down towards the feet, compressing the body to the pont of energetic contact. As I gently push... the body will move beneath my hands until it reaches its compression limit for the amount of pressure I am applying. In doing this I have taken up the slack.

Having engaged the physical body fully, I add slight pressure, which establishes the connection with the energy fields. When I have made good contact with this I just hold the pressure. If there are abnormal waves in that area, I am able to feel the sensations from the person's body in my hands.

Exercise 14. Try to perform this energetic contact, from the shoulders, just as Smith describes it. Take your time, and see what you (and your patient/partner) feel.

Naturally this requires practice to do well. So practise.

Smith states that an evaluation takes him anything from 10 to 30 seconds. This is what you should aim for once you are comfortable with the concepts and your palpatory skills in this area are 'literate'.

How does Smith then balance any abnormal energy waves? He could, he says, override them with a stronger, clearer energy field, or he could introduce a force field which matches the aberrant pattern and hold it, thus allowing the original field to diminish and vanish. A third choice is to make an 'essential connection' with the aberrant pattern and to anchor this as the body tries to pull away.

Whichever he chooses, immediate re-evaluation will often show that the aberration is still present. However, reassessment some days or even weeks later may show that it has normalized. This is not dissimilar to many physical treatment results (trigger points especially) in which changes at the time of treatment may be apparent but minimal, the majority of change taking place later, as homoeostatic mechanisms accomplish their self-regulating tasks.

Smith illustrates his ideas with clinical examples. In one instance he examined a patient who had been in pain since an automobile accident over a year before, in which no significant injury had occurred apart from bruising. Smith was unable to find any cause for the pain until he noted a strong twisting force in the energy field from the right side of the chest to his left abdomen. This represented the twisting force exerted at the time of the accident.

He used traction on the legs to 'engage' this force field (an alternative to the method mentioned previously of pushing down through the shoulders to engage it) and exerted a slightly stronger force field through his body, noting, 'A sensation of a rebounding effect along the energy imprint itself. By anchoring the new field I allowed the rebound to subside.'

A gradual release of first the energy body and then the physical body, and a subsequent resting of the legs on the table, left the patient with a sense of well-being and quietness. Two days later on examination he was free of pain and there were no twisting currents to be found. A number of zero balancing sessions may be needed if greater degrees of imprinting of forces exist.

Exercise 15. Introduce traction from the ankles until slack has been taken out. Hold this, with just a fraction more force, so that the energy field is engaged. What do you feel?

Hold the position and use any of the approaches Smith suggests if you sense a 'lengthening' of the field and a subsequent 'still point', or 'retraction'.

Take care and concentrate.

In palpating areas of trauma Smith tells us of variations in patterns we may expect to palpate, depending upon the type of trauma a patient experienced, specifically detailing ancient Chinese distinctions between 'horse kick injury' and 'camel kick injury'. The first, involving hard hooves, results in local physical trauma, severe at the onset, with healing after days or weeks. The second, involving softer camel hooves, results in mild initial reaction with increasing symptoms as time passes, as the injury 'moves deeper'. It is as though the 'soft' injury fails to stimulate defence mechanisms and therefore disperses through the body/mind/energy fields of the person with subsequent symptoms emerging.

Smith makes an important statement when he says: 'Energetic connections can be lost if our thoughts drift or we are focussed elsewhere. Energy follows thought.' Upledger makes very similar pronouncements, as do most workers in the 'energy field', and this is something the beginner may find useful. When results don't come, ask yourself where your attention was.

Tissue Memory   Upledger reports evidence showing that decerebrate laboratory rats are able to solve food-orientated maze problems, indicating a 'memory' and decision-making facility within the spinal cord. He also reports studies indicating a degree of 'decision making' taking place in the hands of a musician without CNS input. He suggests, 'Perhaps these powers develop in these peripheral locations, in response to a person's need to develop certain skills.'

Upledger employs techniques such as somatoemotional release in which emotional 'scars' are dealt with, and he, along with Smith (see above), holds to the concept that palpable changes occur in the energy fields of the body related to physical, chemical and emotional trauma.

Is this physiologically possible? Professor Irvin Korr, a physiologist of international stature, enters this controversial arena, albeit on a neurological rather than an energy level. In an article 'Somatic dysfunction, osteopathic manipulative treatment and the nervous system' (*Journal of the American Osteopathic Association*, February 1986) Korr states:

Spinal reflexes can be conditioned by repetition or prolongation of given stimulus. According to the hypothesis, like the brain, the cord can learn and remember new behaviour patterns. Whether the (memory) once recorded, needs reinforcement by some kind of afferent stimulation is an open question.

On the influence of somatic changes on the mind he says:

Clinical experience indicates that somatic dysfunction (and manipulation) are powerful influences on brain function and on the perceptions and even the personality of the patient. This experience... raises many fundamental questions and exciting clinical implications.

So Korr seems to be supporting both the idea of a 'memory' independent of the brain as well as of tissue changes (from whatever cause) having a continual impact on 'perceptions and personality' factors. To conclude this survey of opinions, let us look at what Hans Selye M.D., the premier researcher into stress, said on the subject:

The lasting bodily changes (in structure or chemical composition) which underlie effective adaptation or the collapse of it, are after effects of stress; they represent tissue-memories which affect our future somatic behaviour during similar stressful situations. They can be stored.

(The Stress of Life)

Speransky, the great Russian researcher, not only hypothesized such a state of affairs, he also proved it and showed how to reverse it. He stated:

Chemical and infectual trauma of nerve structures result in nervous dystrophy, this, in turn, gives the impulses for the development in the tissue of other pathological change, including those of an inflammatory character. Their disposition at the periphery can be predicted by us in advance, and their boundaries remain unchanged often throughout long periods.

(A Basis for the Theory of Medicine)

Rollin Becker D.O. (see below) reports that Speransky changed these imprinted messages by 'manually flushing or washing the CNS with the animal's or human's own CSF, and the disabled condition in the peripheral tissues normalized'.

Becker himself declares:

Memory reactions occur within the CNS system in all traumatic cases... An area of the body that has been seriously hurt is going to send thousands of sensory messages into the spinal cord segments and brain areas that supply that part of the body. If the injury is severe, or long lasting, these messages will be imprinted into the nervous system similar to imprinting a message on a tape recorder.

Thus the tissues, and the nervous system 'remember' the injury and its pattern of dysfunction long after healing has occurred. It becomes 'facilitated' to that pattern long after the trauma. Finding the eye of the hurricane, the still-point, is the formula which Smith, Upledger and Becker advocate if we are to quieten those aberrant patterns of energy which exist after trauma or misuse.

The brilliant research of Bjorn Nordenstrom M.D. is outlined below. This former Chief of Diagnostic Radiation at the famed Karolinska Institute in Stockholm, has shown that there exists a previously unsuspected energy system which could help to explain the work of researchers such as Smith and Becker.

However, before examining his research results we should investigate the dedicated studies and palpatory techniques of Rollin Becker D.O. (*1963 Yearbook Academy of Applied Osteopathy*, *1964 Yearbook of AOO*, *1965 Yearbook of AAO*) and Alan Becker, D.O. (*1973 Yearbook of AOO* 'Parameters of Resistance').

Becker's Diagnostic Touch   According to Rollin Becker, when a practitioner is first faced by any patient 'The patient is intelligently guessing as to the diagnosis, the physician is scientifically guessing as to the diagnosis, but the patient's body *knows* the problem and is outpicturing it in the tissues.'

Learning to read what the body has to say is the necessary task of diagnosis, and much of this depends upon palpation. 'The first step in developing depth of feel and touch is to re-evaluate the patient from the standpoint, just what does the patient's body want to tell you?' Having set aside the patient's opinions and your initial diagnosis:

> Place your hands and fingers on the patient in the area of his complaint or complaints. Let the feel of the tissues from the inner core of their depths come through to your touch and read, and 'listen' to their story. To get this story it is necessary to know something about potency... and something about the fulcrum.

'Potency' and 'fulcrum' are two areas which we must examine closely as we learn of Becker's remarkable palpatory method. *Potency* tells us the degree, the power of strength, of whatever is being discussed; it also, Becker reminds us, speaks to the ability to control or influence, something. The diagnostic tool which Becker will teach us to use, as we learn to read and understand potency, is the fulcrum, in which the fingers and hands create a condition in which potency becomes apparent.

Becker asks us to acknowledge that 'At the very core of total health there is a potency within the human body manifesting itself in health. At the core of every traumatic or disease condition within the human body is a potency manifesting its interrelationship with the body in trauma and disease. It is up to us to learn to feel this potency.'

He likens this concept to the eye of a hurricane, which carries the potency, or power, of the whole storm. In just this way, within each trauma or disease pattern there is an 'eye' 'within or without the patient' which carries in itself the potency to manifest the condition. This 'eye' is a point of stillness, the existence of which he asks you to accept as you take the time to develop a sense of touch which can perceive it.

The *fulcrum* is a support, or point of support, on which a lever turns in raising or moving something, therefore being a means of exerting pressure or influence. Lief used the term fulcrum to describe the still-resting state of the fingers as the thumb moved towards them in its searching mode in NMT methodology. Smith uses the term fulcrum to describe a 'balance' point via which the therapist 'gets in touch' with the energy body. It is established once the 'slack has been taken out' of the tissues, and an interface created. Becker suggests that his fulcrum should be understood as a 'still-leverage' junction, which may be shifted from place to place, all the while retaining its leverage function.

The would-be palpator achieves this by placing his/her hand(s) near the site complained of by the patient. A fulcrum is then established using the elbow, forearm, crossed fingers, or other convenient area as a supporting point (the fulcrum) allowing the contacting fingers/hand(s) to be gently yet firmly molded to the tissues. The fulcrum provides the working point, free to move if needed, yet stable as the palpation proceeds.

An example is given in which a supine patient with a low back problem is to be examined. The operator sits beside the patient, placing a hand under the sacrum, fingers extended cephalid, and the elbow of that hand resting either on the table or in the operator's own knees. 'By leaning comfortably on his/her elbow, the physician establishes a fulcrum from which to read the changes taking place in the back.' It is the elbow which is the fulcrum.

By applying increased pressure at the fulcrum, causing a slight degree of compression at the sacrum, the operator will 'initiate a kinetic energy that will allow the structure-function of the stress area to begin its pattern to be reflected back to his/her touch'.

If the other hand were similarly placed, under the low back, the fulcrum could be the edge of the table, against which the forearm rests (or an elbow on the knee). Either or both fulcrums may be employed to feel 'the tug of the tissues deep within'.

The operator will also become aware, says Becker, of '*a quiet point, a still-point, an area of stillness within the stress pattern, that is the point of potency of that particular strain*'. He makes it clear that he is discussing the kinetics of the energy fields that make up the stress pattern, and not anatomical/physiological units of tissue when he describes the point of potency.

Exercise 16. Palpate a sacrum using Becker's fulcrum, as described above. Compare this with the sensations noted when using Upledger's sacral assessment.

What is the form of energy being assessed here? Becker doesn't know, and says that it no more matters that we know than that we need to know the nature of electricity before being able to safely use it. This thought has been found to be deeply satisfying to those practitioners, aware of the effectiveness of these ideas and methods, who are unable to accept the Upledger/Smith/chakra/accupuncture models of 'energy'.

Is there any other model? It would be appropriate at this point to

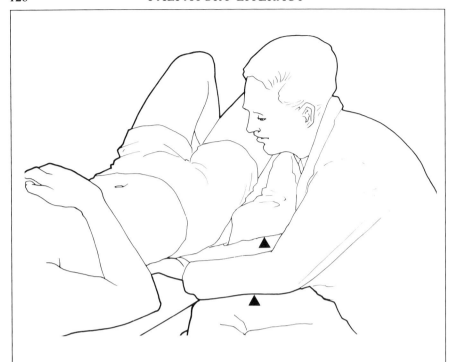

Fig. 19: Low back palpation. Hands under sacrum and low back applies no pressure – contact only. Forearm resting on edge of table acts as Becker's Fulcrum. Increased pressure downwards at the fulcrum palpator's awareness of tissue status.

bring in Dr Nordenstrom's research results, since they may answer the question as to what the form of energy being palpated represents. Nordenstrom, formerly chair of the Karolinska Nobel Assembly, which selects Nobel prize winners in medicine, is hardly a rebel, or maverick. His discoveries are, however, revolutionary. He described his results in his book *Biologically Closed Electric Circuits: Clinical, Experimental and Theoretical Evidence for an Additional Circulatory System.*

It was when using a small spot X-ray technique, in order to define breast and lung tumours, that he first noted an unusual zone around some tumours. He called this a 'corona', and decided to investigate the phenomenon as there was no histological evidence of change in these tissues. By inserting fine needles into these tissues he demonstrated an electric flow, continuing his research on humans and animals, alive and dead, before developing a series of principles.

The first was that energy conversion in tissues over a biologically closed electric circuit can be defined as a fluctuation in electrical potential in a limited area, resulting from injury, tumour and healing. He found that there was an electric flow in tissues which followed selected pathways and that large blood vessels function as insulated electricity conducting cables. He also demonstrated that biologically closed electric circuits produce magnetic changes around an area which can be measured from a distance.

Nordenstrom also discovered that biological factors which cause cancer, of a chemical or physical nature, have the ability to polarize tissues and that therefore 'inactivated biologically closed electric circuits' may represent a common factor in carcinogenesis. He was able to show that there exist differences in electrical potential over an area of a few millimetres around injured (or malignant) tissues.

Is this electricity the energy Smith and Becker are feeling? Are polarizations and fluctuations what is being palpated in an energy cyst? What Nordenstrom has proved is that there is another circulation in the body, that of electricity (or energy) and that it changes measurably in response to disease or injury. It can be assessed by machine, and probably therefore by palpation.

Reviewing this book in *The D.O.* (September 1988) Martyn Richardson D.O. states:

> I had a chemistry professor in college who demonstrated that the molecule consisted of atoms, which consisted of electrons, protons and neutrons, which were not 'solid matter' but electric charges. Therefore everything was nothing – except a collection of electric charges.

Clyde Ford D.C. (*Where Healing Waters Meet*, Station Hill Press, New York 1989) explains a different energy research study which evolved from the simple observation of a chiropractor I.N. Toftness, that skin drag occurred on palpation of 'problem areas'.

His research showed that microwave emissions emanating from the body could be measured, that these varied in relation to areas of excess or diminished activity, and also that they changed after sustained light pressure was applied to such areas.

> Toftness used light pressure to manipulate the body and had a wealth of clinical studies to document the effectiveness of this method. To this he now added the ability to objectively monitor the human electromagnetic field and demonstrate its relationship to the physical condition of the human body. Typically the radiometer detected abnormally high or abnormally low microwave readings in problem areas of the body. After sustained light pressure, these peaks and valleys normalized – the high readings were reduced and the low readings raised. Monitoring the electromagnetic field produced by the body is a unique form of diagnosis because it is truly non-invasive.

Clearly this 'electromagnetic' or microwave transmission from body tissues is a strong contender for what Smith and Becker (and the others we have discussed) are palpating when they speak of 'energy'.

Whatever Becker is palpating, it is obviously significant, and worthy of our learning to do the same.

How long does it take to make an assessment using Becker's methods? Less than 10 minutes is necessary to identify the focal point of potency, he says, and with practice it becomes possible to date old strains (are they weeks, months or years old?) and to tell the difference between the energy patterns of these and those found with 'new' strains. The following exercise which Rollin Becker describes is well worth attempting several times until the principles he is teaching become clear.

Exercise 17.
Stage 1: First sit facing a patient/model who is seated on the edge of a treatment table. Place your hands around the knee, fingers interlocked in the popliteal space. Try to sense as much as you can about the knee applying a compression force towards the hip to see what you can tell about that area. You may get some information, but not much.

Stage 2: Now adopt the same contact with the knee, but this time rest your own elbows on your knees as you do so. Apply the same compression towards the hips and assess what you feel, *using the fulcrum points.*

Becker describes what you might feel this time:

> Feel how the innate natural forces within the thigh and pelvis want to turn the acetabulum either into an internal rotation or an external rotation position. Note the quality and quantity of that turning. Note that if you lean lightly on your elbow fulcrum points you get a more superficial reading from the tissues under your hands even though your hands and interlaced fingers remain light in their control.
>
> Note that if you then lean more firmly on your elbow fulcrum points you get a deeper and deeper impression from the tissues under examination.

The depth of perception is dependent on the firmness of the fulcrum contacts, *not on the firmness of the examining finger contacts.* If there exists a deep strain in the tissues, it is the fulcrum pressure which is increased in order to reach these tissues and their patterns of dysfunction.

This can be done anywhere by the simple expedient of creating a fulcrum under the tissues to be examined, establishing a fulcrum point and tuning in to the information waiting to be uncovered. There are two important riders to this though, says Becker. You must know your anatomy and physiology in order to make sense of the information, and you must divorce yourself from any sense of 'doing'. Just let the story come through. The fulcrum points are listening posts only.

And yet this is not quite the case. For Becker does ask that there be an introduction of a slight compression force, or traction, not in order to actively test the tissues but to 'activate already existing forces within the patient's body'. The example of the pressure towards the acetabulum is useful, for having applied this it would be the innate tendency to externally and internally rotate which would then be palpated. Becker is asking for contact with the 'interface' which Smith described, and the 'still point' which Upledger described, in different terms perhaps, but in essence in much the same manner.

What he adds is the concept of being able to gain deeper perception of, and access to, tissue (or energy) states by use of the fulcrum. Becker calls this diagnostic touch:

It is a form of palpation that one might call an alert observational type of awareness for the functions and dysfunctions from within the patient, utilizing the motive deep energy, deep within the tissues themselves. It is not the patient voluntarily turning the acetabulum but his tissues within the acetabulum turning it for you to observe.

What should you feel as the body's forces play around the fulcrum?

To the outside observer watching our work, our hands are apparently lying quietly on the patient, but the motion, the mobility, the motility we sense from within the patient is considerable, depending on the problem. There is a deliberate pattern that the tissues go through in demonstrating the strain that is within them. Kinetic-energy-wise, they work their way through to a point at which all sense of motion or mobility seems to cease. This is the point of stillness. Even though it is still it is endowed with biodynamic power.

This then is the point of potency within the strain pattern, the still point in this functioning unit which changes as the contact is held, following which a new pattern emerges, and is felt. Normality has been encouraged, or achieved.

Upledger describes the 'interference waves' which result from restriction lesions or trauma. These waves superimpose on normal physiological body motions. Once you identify where the interference waves are coming from the source of the problem is found. Symmetrical placement (gently) of your hands on the head, thoracic inlet, inferior costal margins, pelvis, thighs and feet of the patient allows your hands to perceive the arcs or inherent wave patterns. If these are symmetrical all is well. If the arcs are asymmetrical then you are asked to visualize the radii of these arcs and to determine where they interact. That will be the location of the lesion (restriction or trauma). You need to place your hands on as many sites as necessary to pick up the information required to make this assessment. It is as if there were an infinite number of concentric globes around the lesion, each vibrating and describing arcs. Where is the centre of all the concentric globes? The closer you get, the smaller are the arcs.

Hands may be placed, one on the anterior, one on the posterior surface of the body; both hands will describe arcs, which you should evaluate in order to find a point of intersection. This gives the depth of the lesion. This is Upledger's way of finding 'the eye of the hurricane'. When you have performed a number of Becker's exercises (below) and you come to Exercise 28, try comparing the methods of Upledger and Becker (as well as Smith). One of these may well suit you better than the others, something you can only discover by trying them all.

Rollin Becker gives a series of examples in which he palpates different body regions and describes his contact and fulcrum points. It is suggested that all of these be used in any sequence, on appropriate patients/partners, selecting if possible areas where there is, or has been dysfunction or pathology, so that variations in what is perceived can be observed and learned from. Take as much time as possible.

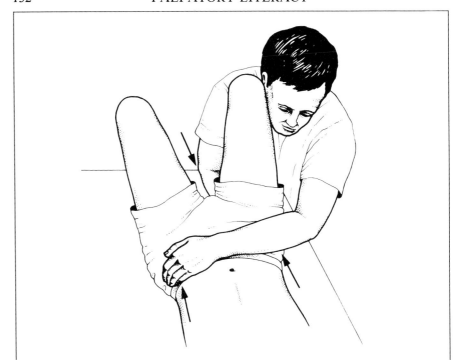

Fig. 20: Palpation of sacrum and pelvis. Becker's fulcrum points are the right elbow on table and contacts on anterior-iliac spines with left hand/arm.

Exercise 18. To assess the sacrum and pelvis. Have the patient supine, knees flexed. Sit on a stool of appropriate height on the patient's right side, facing the head, and place your right hand under the sacrum, finger tips on spinous processes of 5th lumbar vertebrae. Your right elbow rests on the table as the fulcrum. Your left hand and arm bridge the anterior superior spines of the ilium so that either the left hand on the left ASIS or the left elbow on the right ASIS can act as fulcrums if pressure is applied through them. The physician may alternate his use of one or the other ASIS as a fulcrum point in examining the opposite ilium in its functioning relationship with the sacrum. The pelvis and its relationships with the sacrum, lumbar spine and hips below can all be assessed. It is particularly useful for assessment of sacral involvement of whiplash injuries.

Exercise 19. To assess sacrum/ilio-sacrum and low lumbar. Have the patient in the same position as 18 above, with one hand under the sacrum as above, same fulcrum point. The other hand lies under the ilio-sacral articulation, finger tips on the lower lumbar spinous processes. That hand's fulcrum is on your crossed knee, or on the edge of the table. In this position low back and sacroiliac dysfunction can be assessed and treated 'using the forces within the problem'.

Exercise 20. Assessment of psoas and upper lumbar problems. The examining (cephalid) hand is under the supine patient's lumbar spine, fulcrum point on operator's crossed knees. The other hand and arm (caudad) bridge the patient's drawn up knees. Light compression on the fulcrum point allows assessment of superficial lumbar strains. Increased compression on the fulcrum point allows assessment of psoas. Compression of the acetabulae by pressing through the knees towards the hips, further activates the psoas while it is being examined.

Exercise 21. Assessment of lower thorax. Operator sits at head of table with hands under supine patient's upper back at level of insertion of trapezius, bilaterally (mid-thoracic area). Elbows/ forearms are fulcrum, resting on the table. Information from this area is combined with that gained in previous assessment, above.

Exercise 22. Assessment of upper thorax. Seated at head of patient (head on pillow) one hand slides under the pillow and rests against the upper thoracic spinous processes, fingers fanned out to contact ribs as well. Elbow is fulcrum point. The other hand rests on the sternum. The elbow of that arm can also find a fulcrum, on the patient's pillow.

Becker reports that ideally the sternum should move dorsally (i.e. towards the spine) on inhalation and ventrally (towards the ceiling)

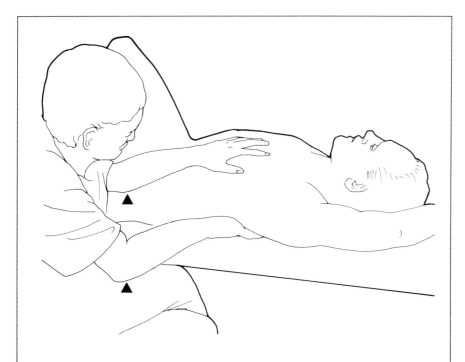

Fig. 21: Palpation of rib cage. Becker's fulcrums are on the operator's crossed knees and patient's anterior superior iliac spine (left).

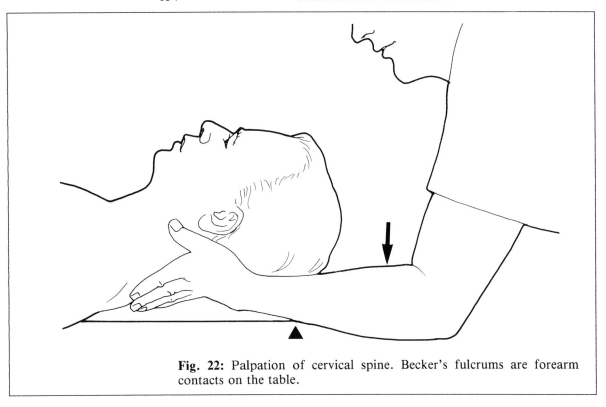

Fig. 22: Palpation of cervical spine. Becker's fulcrums are forearm contacts on the table.

on exhalation. It is common for the normal pattern to be achieved after this 'palpation'.

'Upper thoracic strains are readily found (and easily corrected) in this position, using biodynamic and biokynetic forces and potencies within the patient.'

Exercise 23. To assess the rib cage. The operator sits to the side of the supine patient, the caudad hand lies under the rib cage with fingertips resting just beyond the spinous processes. The fulcrum point is on the operator's crossed knees. The other hand rests on the anterior ends of the same ribs, fulcrum point being the forearm which rests on the patient's ASIS. A slight compression at the fulcrum points initiates motion at the heads of the ribs being examined, allowing strains to be evaluated and treated. The entire rib cage can be assessed, the hands changing position as needed.

Exercise 24. Palpation of the liver. The operator sits on the left side of the supine patient, caudal hand under the lower ribs, fulcrum point on crossed knee. The other hand rests over the liver, spanning the lower costal border. Pressure through the fulcrum point allows biodynamic and biokinetic (disturbed) forces to be felt and assessed.

Exercise 25. Assessment of cervical spine. Operator is at head of supine patient with hands bilaterally bridging the entire cervical region from the base of the skull (hypothenar eminence contacts here) to the upper thorax, where the fingertips lie. The fulcrum points are the forearms which lie on the table. General assessment is possible in this position and individual segments can be localized by finger contact.

Exercise 26. Assessment of occipto-atlantal articulation. Operator sits in same position as for Exercise 25. Base of skull rests on palm of hand, fingers curved upwards to contact posterior tubercle of atlas. The forearm rests on the table as a fulcrum point. The other hand rests on the vertex of the head bringing it into slight forward bending on the neck to facilitate the other hand's contact. Pressure on the fulcrum brings strain patterns into palpable view.

Exercise 27. Assessment of basilar area of skull. Operator's hands are lightly interlaced, with patient's head resting on them, thumbs lie superior to ears extending towards face. The forearms on the table are the fulcrum points. Very slight compression through the fulcrum allows assessment to begin.

Alan Becker D.O., in 'Parameters of Resistance' (*Academy of Applied Osteopathy* September 1973) discusses engrained patterns which we all carry – in much the same way as computers which have been programmed – whether these allow normal or abnormal function. In assessment and treatment he carries Rollin Becker's 'diagnostic touch' concepts further, stating:

> I make contact with the involved tissues and apply enough pressure to get the patient's attention and to initiate the automatic response. Then I ask the patient to close his eyes and look at my fingers, to be aware of what is happening to his body. By this means I persuade him to take conscious control of the program and re-evaluate his standards of normal, acceptable and tolerable data. Then as I lead the structures towards increased ease and balance, the patient senses the changes and tends either to install new action programs which include the new data or to re-establish the ones which were in effect before abnormal data was encouraged.

In discussing a whiplash injury he illustrates this, saying:

> The problem is complicated by the fact that the body has been subjected to forces that entered it in a direction that crosses the normal direction of movement. Such forces tend to produce wavelike movement within the fluid cells of the body, and the inertia of the body, which is trying to continue whatever programs are in action at the time, causes a counterwave directed towards the point of impact.

These two forces set up a wave-like pattern, a ridge of energy, a built-in distortion around which the defensive patterns are built. These have to be removed by dissipation of the energy rather than by force. Only then, Becker insists, can new, more appropriate, patterns be established by the patient. The resistance of built-in patterns, whether these relate to habit or to injury, is something the palpating practitioner should be acutely aware of, for this is a key feature of the territory being explored.

Here we enter the area of structural reintegration, postural re-education, Alexander technique, Feldenkreis' work and other methods which require a relearning of how we use ourselves. Becker's contribution seems to be that he calls on a conscious awareness from the patient as Rollin Becker's approach is applied, in order to have them become aware of the changes which are taking place, and to have them support and encourage these.

> **Exercise 28.** The final exercise in this section asks you to incorporate at one time the concepts of Upledger, Smith and Rollin Becker, as you palpate the motions of CSF, energy and other intrinsic expressions of function in various areas of your patient/partner. Move from the methods of Smith to those of Becker and back again.
>
> Which gives you the most information? Which do you feel more comfortable with? Do you now agree that tissue has a memory?

Are these exercises likely to be of value in a clinical setting? Dr Philip Greenman (*Principles of Manual Medicine*) discussing myofascial release technique, a subtle yet extremely clinical tool, states:

> This [myofascial release] is directed towards a biomechanical effect and a neurophysiological effect. Ward has coined a mnemonic: $POE(T^2)$. POE stands for point of entry into the musculoskeletal system. Entry may be from the lower extremity, the upper extremity, through the thoracic cage, through the abdomen, or from the cranial cervical juntion. The two Ts stand for traction and twist. In most of the techniques traction produces stretch along the long axis of the myofascial elements that are shortened and tightened. The stretch should always be applied in the long axis rather than transversely across myofascial elements. Introduction of a twisting force provides the opportunity to localize the traction, not only at the point of contact with the patient, but also at points some distance away.

He suggests that beginners try to develop the ability to sense change in the freedom or restriction of tissues, some distance from the point which is being contacted. Thus if the ankles are being grasped and traction introduced, an attempt should be made to feel 'through the extremities' to the knee, hip, sacroiliac joint up into the spine itself. Concentration and practice can allow this skill to develop.

In his text Dr Greenman describes exercises which will allow the practitioner to develop the skills necessary to perform myofascial release techniques. These involve palpation of a body area, starting from above the skin, moving to a light contact which attempts 'to sense the inherent movement of the patient's tissues under your hand' (an 'inherent oscillation').

The first step then is to master the ability to apply pressure, or make contact, without movement, followed by being able to palpate the motions which are constantly at work within the tissue without influencing them. This is precisely what the various exercises given in this chapter should allow you to do.

Greenman gives a concluding exercise, palpation of the motion of the sacrum, with the patient first supine and then prone. This you should by now be able to perform. And as he says: 'When you have been able to identify inherent soft tissue and bony movement you are well on your way to being able to use myofascial release technique.'

Hopefully the methods described above, based on the work of these marvellous researchers into human physiology, will allow greater skill in our endeavours.

The Morphology of Reflex (and Acupuncture) Points

Melzack and Wall (*The Challenge of Pain*) have shown that at least 75 per cent of trigger points are acupuncture points, according to the traditional meridian maps. The rest are 'honorary' acupuncture points since, according to Traditional Chinese Medicine, all spontaneously tender areas (whether or not they lie on the meridians) are suitable for acupuncture (or acupressure) treatment, and a trigger point is nothing if it is not spontaneously tender.

Recent evidence using thermographic imaging has shown that the actual size of a trigger point is fairly small, approximately 2 millimetres in diameter, rather than the previously suggested 5 to 10 millimetres (Peter Diakow D.C. 'Thermographic Imaging of Myofascial Trigger Points' *Journal of Manipulative and Physiological Therapeutics* 11: 2; 1988). Their incidence in young adults is shown to be 54 per cent in females and 45 per cent in males (age group 35 to 50). If they usually lie in the same place as acupuncture points, what tissues are involved?

Professor Jean Bossy, of the Faculty of Medicine, University of Montpellier, in France has examined the tissues extensively ('Morphological data concerning acupuncture points and channel networks' *Acupuncture and ElectroTherapeutics Research International Journal* 9, 1984). He informs us that all motor points of medical electrology are acupuncture points (which he calls 'privileged loci of the organism which allow exchanges between the inner body and the environment'). Head's maxima points, Hackett's points, visceral points, the chakra points – all are acupuncture points. He sizes them even smaller than Diakow, at between 1 and 5 millimetres in diameter. The skin manifestation is, he says, 'easier to feel than to see. The most superficial morphological expression is a cupule.'

And under the skin (which is a little thinner than surrounding skin) of these (privileged loci), there are common features. Neurovascular bundles are commonly found, and connective tissue is always a feature, with fatty tissue sometimes present. Vessels and nerves seem to be important common features, although their stimulation during treatment is usually indirect, as the result of deformation of connective tissue and consequent traction.

In some instances, tendons, periarticular structures, or muscle tissues are involved, as part of the acupuncture/trigger point morphology. However, after extensive dissection, Bossy avers that, 'Fat and connective tissue are determinants for the appearance of the acupuncture sensation (*De qi*).'

Thus it seems that effective reflex effects only occur 'through the stimulation of multiple and various anatomical structures'. The most useful information which this study provides is that, on palpation, a slight 'cupule' or depression, overlayed with slightly thinner skin tissue, can be felt, and that this indicates an acupuncture point (which if sensitive is 'active', and quite likely to also be a trigger point). As we have seen in Chapter 3, other palpatory signs exist, skin 'drag', and loss of elastic qualities being the most important palpatory indications of active reflex activity.

Chapter 6

Assessment of 'Abnormal Mechanical Tension' in the Nervous System

We will shortly be examining some extremely important assessment techniques for abnormal tension in neural structures. Before doing so it is necessary to look at some of the potential implications, other than pain, which such tensions hold. We need therefore to briefly examine one physiological component which may be involved: the trophic function of nerves.

Irvin Korr Ph.D., the primary researcher into the neurological and pathophysiological processes involved in osteopathic medicine over the past half century, has studied the phenomenon of the transport and exchange of macromolecular materials along neural pathways. Among his pertinent (to our study) findings are that the influence of nerves on target organs and muscles depends largely on delivery of specific neuronal proteins. There is also evidence of a return pathway by means of which messenger substances are transferred back from target organs to the central nervous system and brain.

In one of Korr's examples (*Spinal Cord as Organizer of Disease Processes*, Part 4, 'Axonal transport and neurotrophic function in relation to somatic dysfunction', March 1981, *Academy of Applied Osteopathy* pp.451–58) it is shown that red and white muscles, which differ morphologically, functionally and chemically, can have all these differences reversed if their innervation is 'crossed', so that red muscles receive white muscle innervation and vice versa. 'This means, in effect that the nerve instructs the muscle what kind of muscle to be, and is an expression of a neurally mediated genetic influence.'

In other words it is the nerve which determines which genes in a muscle will be suppressed and which expressed, and this information is carried in the material being transported along the axons. When a muscle loses contact with its nerve (anterior poliomyelitis for example) atrophy occurs, not as a result of disuse but because of the loss of the integrity of the connection between nerve cells and muscle cells at the myoneural junction, where nutrient exchange occurs irrespective of whether or not impulses are being transmitted.

These and other functions depend upon the flow of axonally transported proteins, phospholipids, glycoproteins, neurotransmitters and their precursors, enzymes, mitochondria and other organelles. The rate of transport of such substances varies from 1mm/day to several hundred mm/day, with 'different cargoes being carried at different rates'. Korr reports that 'The motor powers (for the waves of transportation) are provided by the axon itself.'

Retrograde transportation seems to be 'a fundamental means of communication between neurons and between neurons and non-neuronal cells'. Korr believes this process to have an important role in maintenance of 'the plasticity of the nervous system, serving to keep motor-neurons and muscle cells, or two synapsing neurons, mutually adapted to each other and responsive to each other's changing circumstances'.

What are the clinical implications of this knowledge and, more specifically, how is this related to our study of palpation? We certainly ought to understand what influences are operating on the tissues we palpate. For example, knowledge of the craniosacral rhythmic fluid fluctuations, and of the tubular structure of collagen fibrils which transport CSF, gives us an awareness of what we might be feeling as we palpate for these rhythms.

Similarly awareness of the trophic influence of neural structures on the structural and functional characteristics of soft tissues carries at least as much importance, especially when we realize just how vulnerable these nutrient highways are to disruption:

> Any factor which causes derangement of transport mechanisms in the axon, or that chronically alters the quality or quantity of the axonally transported substances, could cause the trophic influences to become detrimental. This alteration in turn would produce aberrations of structure, function, and metabolism, thereby contributing to dysfunction and disease.

Among the negative influences frequently operating on these transport mechanisms, Korr informs us, are 'deformations of nerves and roots, such as compression, stretching, angulation and torsion'. These stresses occur all too often in humans, says Korr, and are particularly likely where neural structures are most vulnerable:

> In their passage over highly mobile joints, through bony canals, intervertebral foramina, fascial layers, and tonically contracted muscles (for example posterior rami of spinal nerves and spinal extensor muscles).

Korr further amplifies his concern over negative influences on neural trophic function when he discusses 'sustained hyperactive peripheral neurons (sensory, motor and autonomic)'.

For when there is a high rate of discharge from neural structures (facilitated segments and trigger points, for example) the metabolism of neurons are affected, 'and almost certainly their synthesis and turnover of proteins and other macromolecules'. These thoughts (and others of Korr's given below) on the vital trophic role of the nervous system, over and above its conduction of impulses, should be borne in mind as we examine methods of assessing adverse mechanical tension in the nervous system.

Assessment of Adverse Mechanical Tension (AMT) in the Nervous System

Testing for, and treating, 'tensions' in neural structures offers us an alternative method for dealing with some forms of pain and dysfunction, since such adverse mechanical tension is often a major component cause of musculoskeletal dysfunction as well as more widespread pathology (bear Korr's research in mind).

Maitland (*Vertebral Manipulation*) suggests that we consider this form of assessment and treatment to involve 'mobilization' of the neural structures, rather than simply stretching them. He and others recommended that these methods be reserved for conditions which fail to respond adequately to normal mobilization of soft and osseous structures (muscles, joints and so on). Maitland and Butler (see below) have over the years discussed those mechanical restrictions which impinge on neural structures in the vertebral canals and elsewhere.

Recently, Butler and Gifford (*Physiotherapy*, November 1989) taking Maitland's concepts further, have outlined a series of 'Base Tests' which can be used to discover precise mechanical restrictions relating to the nervous system. The five 'Base (Tension) Tests' which will be described are useful not only for diagnosis but for passive mobilization of the structures involved. The tissues involved in 'mechanical tension' often include the nerve itself, as well as its surrounding muscle, connective tissue, circulatory structures, dura and so on. The Five Tension Test methods used are:

- Straight Leg Raising (SLR).
- Prone Knee Bending (PNB).
- Passive Neck Flexion (PNF).
- A combination of these called 'Slump' position.
- The upper limb tension test (ULTT).

These tests are often performed in conjuction with each other (for example 'slump' together with PNB). Despite some of these tests being familiar in other settings, if reliable results are wanted it is vital that the methodology for their use, as described in this particular context, be followed closely. Butler and Gifford report that studies have shown that changes in tension in lumbar nerve roots have been demonstrated during PNF, and that there is often an instant alteration in neck and arm (and sometimes head) pain via the addition of ankle dorsiflexion during SLR. The additional stretches, such as ankle dorsiflexion during SLR, are described in this work as 'sensitizing' manoeuvres.

The Butler/Gifford approach calls for careful positioning of the region being tested, as changes in pain are assessed, as well as the use of these passive stretches as a means of inducing release of restrictions when they are discovered. The developers of Tension Tests for adverse mechanical tension in the nervous system point out that *body movements (and therefore these tests) not only produce an increase in tension within the nerve but also move the nerve in relation to surrounding tissues.*

The surrounding tissues have been called the mechanical interface (MI). These adjacent tissues are those which can move independently of the nervous system (e.g. supinator muscle is the MI to the radial nerve, as it passes through radial tunnel). Any pathology in the MI can produce abnormalities in nerve movement, resulting in tension on neural structure with unpredictable ramifications. Good examples of MI pathology are nerve impingement by disc protrusion or osteophyte contact, and carpel tunnel constriction. These problems would be regarded as *mechanical* in origin as far as the nerve restriction is concerned. Any symptoms resulting from this sort of (mechanical) problem will be more readily provoked in tests which involve movement rather than pure (passive) tension.

Chemical or inflammatory causes of neural tension also occur, resulting in 'interneural fibrosis' and leading to reduced elasticity and increased 'tension', which would become obvious with tension testing of these structures. (See in Chapter 4 discussion on progression from acute to chronic in soft tissue dysfunction.

Such pathophysiological changes (inflammation, chemical (toxic) damage and so on) often lead on to internal mechanical restrictions (Adverse Mechanical Tensions or AMT) unlike examples such as disc lesions in which an external agency causes this 'tension' (AMT). Adverse Mechanical Tension changes do not necessarily affect nerve conduction, according to Butler and Gifford; however Korr's research shows it to be likely that axonal transport would be affected.

When a tension test is positive (i.e. pain is produced by one or another element of the test – initial position alone or with 'sensitizing' additions) it indicates only that there is some adverse mechanical tension (AMT) somewhere in the nervous system and not that this is necessarily at the site of reported pain.

Butler and Gifford report on research indicating that 70 per cent of 115 patients with either carpel tunnel syndrome, or lesions of the ulnar nerve at the elbow, showed clear electro-physiological and clinical evidence of neural lesions in the neck. This is, they maintain, because of a 'double crush' phenomenon in which a primary, and often longstanding, disorder, perhaps in the spine, results in secondary or 'remote' dysfunction at the periphery. This can also work in reverse, for example where wrist entrapment of the ulnar nerve leads ultimately to nerve entrapment at the elbow (they term this 'reversed double crush').

Let us again refer to Korr's evidence of retrograde transportation of axonal flow, as this is one possible factor influencing such changes. In the book *Physiological Basis of Osteopathic Medicine* he says:

To appreciate the vulnerability of the segmental nervous system to somatic insults it must be understood that much of the pathway taken by nerves as they emerge from the cord is actually through skeletal muscle. The great contractile forces of skeletal muscles with the accompanying chemical changes exert profound influences on the metabolism and excitability of neurons. In this environment the neurons are subject to quite considerable mechanical and chemical influences of various kinds, compression and torsion and many others... slight mechanical stresses may, over a period of time, produce adhesions, constrictions and angulations imposed by protective layers. [Perhaps involving friction protectors such as meningeal extensions including nerve sheaths or nerve sleeves].

Such mechanical stresses also, of course, interfere with axoplasmic flow:

> Flowing down every single nerve fibre is a stream of nerve cell cytoplasm in a volume so great that the nerve is said to 'turn over' its material completely three or four times a day, and this flow is essential to the continual nourishment of the fibres themselves along their entire length.

Since this axoplasmic flow also nourishes target tissues, in addition to which the nerves are known to carry back chemical messages from the tissues towards the cord in the same way, interference with the flow of chemical messages due to increased 'tensions' has major health implications. Korr further elaborated on four types of disturbance of nerve function which can result from local tissue impingement:

1. Increased neural excitability at the point of disturbance;
2. Triggering of supernumerary impulses (frequency of discharge from and into the spinal cord, as well as to the periphery increases, the patterns becoming 'garbled').
3. 'Cross-talk' which occurs when nerve fibres pick up electrical stimuli from neighbouring nerves.
4. Local stresses continually report to the spinal cord, thus 'jamming' normal transmission of patterned feedback.

Butler and Gifford note that certain anatomical areas, where the nervous system moves only a little relative to the surrounding interface during motion, or where the system is relatively fixed, are the most likely regions for AMT to develop. This is often noted where nerves branch or enter a muscle. Such areas are called 'tension points' and these are referred to in the test descriptions:

1. A positive tension test is one in which the patient's symptoms are reproduced by the test procedure *and* where these can be altered by variations in what are termed 'sensitizing manoeuvres' which are used 'to add weight to', and confirm, the initial diagnosis of AMT.

   Adding dorsiflexion during SLR is an example of a sensitizing manoeuvre.
2. Precise symptom reproduction may not be possible, but the test is still possibly relevant if other abnormal symptoms are produced during the test and accompanying sensitizing procedures. Comparison with the test findings on an opposite limb, for example, may indicate an abnormality worth exploring.
3. Altered range of movement is another indicator of abnormality, whether this is noted during the initial test position or during sensitizing additions.

Variations of passive motion of nervous system during examination and treatment:

1. An increase in tension can be produced in the interneural component, where there is tension from both ends, so to speak, as in the 'slump' test.
2. Increased tension can be produced in the extraneural component, which then produces the maximum movement of the nerve in relation to its mechanical interface (such as in SLR) with the likelihood of restrictions showing up at 'tension points'.
3. Movement of extraneural tissues in another plane can be engineered.

1. Straight Leg Raising (SLR)

This should be used in all vertebral disorders, all lower limb disorders and some upper limb disorders.

The leg is raised in the sagittal plane, knee extended.
Sensitizing additions:

- Ankle dorsiflexion (this stresses tibial component of sciatic nerve).
- Ankle plantarflexion plus inversion (this stresses common peroneal nerve, useful in anterior shin and dorsal foot symptoms).
- Passive neck flexion.
- Increased medial hip rotation.
- Increased hip adduction.
- Altered spinal position (example is given of left SLR being 'sensitized' by lateral flexion to the right of the spine).

Note: On SLR there is caudad movement of lumbosacral nerve roots in relation to interfacing tissue (hence there is a 'positive' indication from SLR if prolapsed intervertebral disc exists).

Less well known is the fact that the tibial nerve, proximal to the knee, moves caudad (in relation to MI) during SLR, whereas distal to the knee it moves cranially. There is no movement behind the knee itself, which is therefore known as a 'tension point'. The common peroneal nerve is attached firmly to the head of the fibula (another 'tension point').

2. Prone Knee Bend (PKB)

This test moves nerves and roots from L2, 3, 4 and, particularly, the femoral nerve and its branches.

The knee of the prone patient is flexed while hip and thigh are stabilized or with the patient side-lying and hip in extension (the latter position is thought more appropriate for identifying entrapped lateral femoral cutaneous nerve). PKB stretches rectus femoris and rotates the pelvis forward, thus extending the lumbar spine, which can confuse interpretation of nerve impingement symptoms.

Reliance on sensitizing manoeuvres helps with such interpretation. These include:

- Cervical flexion
- 'Slump' in side-lying posture
- Variations of hip abduction, adduction, rotation.

3. 'Slump Test'

This is regarded by Butler as the most important test in this series. It links neural and connective tissue components from the pons to the feet and requires care in performing and interpreting.

It is suggested for testing in all spinal disorders, most lower limb disorders and some upper limb disorders (especially those which seem to involve the nervous system).

The test involves thoracic and lumbar flexion, followed by cervical flexion, knee extension and ankle dorsiflexion, sometimes with hip flexion (produced by either bringing the trunk forwards on the hips, or by increasing SLR).

Note: Cadaver studies demonstrate that neuromeningeal movement occurs in various directions, with C6, T6 and L4 intervertebral levels being regions of constant state (i.e. no movement, therefore 'tension points'). Butler reports that many restrictions, identified during the 'Slump' test, may only be corrected by appropriate spinal manipulation.

Sensitizing manoeuvres during 'Slump testing' are achieved as a rule by changes in terminal joints. Butler gives examples: should 'slump position' reproduce (for example) lumbar and radiating thigh

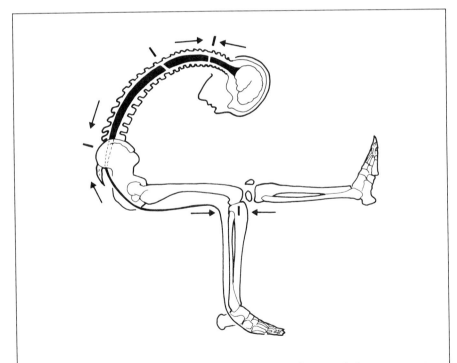

Fig. 23: Slump test position stretches entire neural network from pons to feet. Note direction of stretch of dura mater and nerve roots. As leg comes from position A to B movement of tibial nerve in relation to tibia and femur is indicated by arrows. No neural movement occurs behind the knee or at levels C6. T6 or L4.

pain, a change in head position – say away from full neck flexion – could result in total relief of these symptoms. A change in ankle and knee positions could significantly change cervical, thoracic or head pain.

In both instances this would confirm that AMT was operating, although the site would remain obscure.

The 'slump test' involves tension on the nervous system rather than motion.

Note: Butler points out that SLR is more likely to pick up neural tension in the lumbosacral region. It is possible for SLR to be positive and 'Slump' negative, and vice versa, so both should always be performed. The following findings have been reported in research using the 'slump test':

1. Mid-thoracic to T9 are painful on trunk and neck (50 per cent of 'normal' individuals).
2. Hamstring and posterior knee pain with trunk and neck flexion when knees extended, increasing with ankle dorsiflexion. Restrictions in ankle dorsiflexion during trunk/neck flexion plus knee extension. These signs are considered normal if symmetrical.
3. There is a common decrease in pain noted on release of neck flexion, and an increase in range of knee extension or ankle dorsiflexion, on release of neck flexion.

If patients' symptoms are reproduced by the 'slump' position, and can be relieved by sensitizing manouevres, you have a positive test.

This is further emphasized if, as well as symptom reproduction, there is a symmetrical decrease in range of motion which does not happen when tension is absent. For example, bilateral ankle dorsiflexion is restricted during slump but disappears when the neck is not flexed.

In some instances anomalous reactions are observed in which, for example, pain increases when the neck is taken out of flexion, or when trunk on hip flexion decreases symptoms. Mechanical interface (MI) pathology may account for this. Variations which can be used include the addition of trunk side-bending and rotation or even extension; hip adduction, abduction or rotation; and varying neck positions.

4. Passive Neck Flexion (PNF)
As with SLR this takes up slack from one end only. It allows movement of neuromeningeal tissues in relation to the spinal canal, which is its mechanical interface (MI). 22 per cent of patients with back pain were shown to have a positive PNF test in an industrial survey. Variations such as neck extension, lateral flexion and PNF, in combination with other tests, should be used for screening purposes for AMT.

5. Upper Limb Tension Tests (ULTT)
This test, developed in Australia by physiotherapist Robert Elvey, has

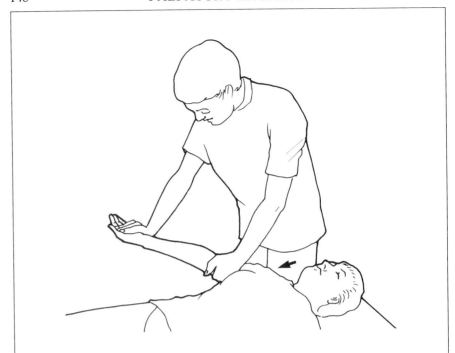

Fig. 24: Upper limb tension test (2).
Note operator's thigh depresses shoulder as arm is placed in maximum
internal rotation of the shoulder, elbow extension and forearm pronation
as hand is also pronated and extended.

been called the 'SLR of the arm'. Use of both ULTTs is suggested in
cases involving thoracic, cervical and upper limb symptoms, even if
this involves only local finger pain. There are two variations:

- ULTT(1) is performed in the sequence of:
  (1) abduction, extension and lateral rotation of the glenohumeral
  joint;
  (2) supination of the forearm and elbow extension;
  (3) wrist and finger extension.
  As this position is held, sensitization is performed by adding
  cervical lateral flexion away from the tested side, or the addition of
  ULTT(1) on the other arm simultaneously, or by use of SLR bi- or
  uni-laterally, or by using pronation rather than supination.
  Note: A great deal of nerve movement occurs during this test. In
  cadavers up to 2 cm movement of the median nerve in relation to its
  MI has been observed during neck and wrist movement. 'Tension
  points' in the upper limb are found at the shoulder and elbow.
- ULTT(2). Butler developed this test and finds it more sensitive than
  ULTT(1). He maintains that it replicates the working posture
  involved in many instances of upper limb repetition disorders
  ('overuse syndrome'). In using ULTT(2) comparison is always
  made with the other arm.

Example of right side ULTT(2):

Patient lies close to right side of couch so that scapula is free of the surface. Trunk and legs are angled towards left foot of bed so that patient feels secure. Operator stands to side of patients head facing feet with left thigh depressing the shoulder girdle. Patient's fully flexed right arm is supported at elbow and wrist by operator's hands. Slight variations in the degree and angle of shoulder depression ('lifted' towards ceiling, held towards floor) may be used, by alteration of thigh contact. Holding the shoulder depressed, operator's right hand grasps patient's right wrist while elbow is held by left hand. With these contacts arm can be taken into internal or external rotation, elbow flexion or extension, forearm supination or pronation.

A combination of shoulder internal rotation, elbow extension and forearm pronation (with shoulder constantly depressed) is considered to offer the most sensitive test position. When an arm position such as this has been adopted the operator slides his right hand down onto the patient's open hand, with thumb between patient's thumb and index finger. Changes such as supination or pronation, stretching of fingers/thumb or radial and ulnar deviations can be introduced in this way with good control.

Sensitization may involve neck movement (sidebend away and so on) or altered shoulder position, such as increased abduction or extension. Cervical lateral flexion away from the tested side causes increased arm symptoms in 93 per cent of people, and cervical lateral flexion towards the tested side increases symptoms in 70 per cent of cases.

Note: Butler reports that ULTT mobilizes the cervical dural theca in a transverse direction (whereas the 'slump' mobilizes the dural theca in an antero-posterior direction as well as longitudinally).

Precautions and contraindications:

1. Take care of spine during 'slump test' if disc problems are involved or if neck is sensitive (or prone to dizziness).
2. Watch neck during side-bending in ULTT.
3. If area is sensitive take care over aggravating existing conditions (arm more likely than leg to be 'stirred up').
4. If obvious neurological problems exist take special care not to exacerbate by vigorous or strong stretching. Similar precautions apply to diabetic, MS, recent surgical patients or where the area being tested is much affected by circulatory deficit.
5. Do not use the tests if there has been recent onset or worsening of neurological signs, or if there is any cauda equina or cord lesion.

It is logical, bearing in mind Korr's evidence as to the many ways in which soft tissue (and osseous) dysfunction can impinge on neural structures, that maximum relaxation of muscle involved in interface tissue should be achieved, by normal methods, before such tests (or subsequent treatment based on such tests) are considered.

It is not within the scope of this text to describe methods for releasing abnormal tensions, except to suggest that, as in (most of) the examples of tests for shortened postural muscles given in Chapter 4, the treatment positions are a replication of the test positions. Butler suggests that in treating adverse mechanical tensions in the nervous system in this way, initial stretching should commence well away from the site of pain in sensitive individuals and conditions.

Re-testing regularly during treatment is also wise, in order to see whether gains in range of motion or lessening of pain provocation during testing are being achieved.

It is critical that any sensitivity provoked by treatment should subside immediately the technique is stopped or there is probable irritation of the neural tissues involved.

Note: The inclusion of descriptions of these (and other) tests, in a text primarily aimed at enhanced palpatory literacy, may be questioned. What have they to do with palpation?

I consider that the testing for muscle length, or strength (not dealt with here as adequate information is readily available on this subject), joint play, and possible adverse mechanical tension in nerves, are all logical extensions of palpation of the skin (and indeed of the region just above the skin) as well as of muscles, fascia and so on.

The concepts of 'end-feel', range of motion, and restrictive barriers are discussed below. Assessment of such barriers and restrictions, as well as normal 'end-feel', requires a delicacy of touch which must be considered to be a major element of palpatory literacy. Furthermore awareness of what Butler calls 'tension' points, should be added to the knowledge we hold in mind, as we palpate and test in other ways than those described above. As we use the methods developed by Lief, Nimmo, Lewit, Beal, Smith or Becker (or any other method of palpation) such knowledge is potentially very useful indeed. If on palpation 'changes' were palpated in such 'tension' point areas, the possibility of nervous system involvement would be clear only if these concepts were understood. Use of one, or other, or all, of the tests described above would then either confirm or deny this possibility. Subsequent use of tests to assess for shortened muscle structures (Chapter 4) and joint restrictions (Chapter 7) would also be appropriate, as such shortening alone could be the cause of adverse tension in the nervous system.

Joint Play/'End-Feel'/Range of Motion: What Are They?

Joint play refers to the particular movements between bones associated with either separation of the surfaces (as in traction), or parallel movement of joint surfaces (also known as translation or translatoric gliding).

Some degree of movement is possible between most joints, restricted only by the degree of soft tissue elasticity. Any change in length of such soft tissues therefore automatically alters the range of joint mobility – also known as the degree of 'slack' – which is available.

In applying traction to a joint (at right angles to the joint surface) a slight separation, merely removing the intrinsic compressive force of surrounding tissues, is known as a Grade I degree of traction. When the 'slack' is removed by further separation, tightening the surrounding tissues, this is a Grade II degree of traction. This increases to a Grade III when actual stretch of the tissues is introduced.

When a gliding translation between joint surfaces occurs this takes place with the surfaces parallel to each other (also called 'roll-gliding'). Only a portion of the joint will be able to move parallel with its opposing surface in this way, at any time, since the surfaces are not flat, only one part being parallel at any moment (due to the surfaces being incongruent).

A Grade I glide involves slack being taken up and a degree of tightening of the soft tissues. Grade II involves actual stretching of these as translation continues.

An important rule relating to whether the joint surface is concave or convex is described by Professor Freddy Kaltenborn in *Mobilization of the Extremity Joints* (Olaf Norlis Bokhandel, Universitetgaten 24, N-0162 Oslo 1, Norway 1985). This states that if a concave surface moves in relation to another surface then the direction of gliding and the direction of the movement of the bone are in the same direction. This means that the moving bone and the concave surface of the joint are on the same side as the axis of motion.

However when a convex joint surface is in a gliding motion the bone movement will be in the opposite direction to the glide. This means that the moving surface and the bone lie on opposite sides of the axis of rotation. Thus, when there is a joint restriction, ascertained by careful assessment of joint play (i.e. gliding) it is essential to know the relative shape of the articulation.

In the case of a convex joint surface (for example head of humerus) the bone will need to be moved by the therapist in a direction opposite to the direction of restricted bone motion in order to increase improved range of motion in the joint.

In the case of a concave joint surface (for example proximal head of ulna) the bone will need to be moved in the same direction as the direction of restriction of bone movement in order to improve range of motion in the joint.

All joints have a 'normal' range of motion, and guidelines as to these are found in Chapter 7. Palpation should involve a screening of these for abnormal restriction or hypermobility.

The end of a range of motion of a joint may be described as having a certain 'feel' and this is called 'end-feel'. If a joint is taken actively or passively to its maximum range of normal motion it reaches its *physiological barrier*. This has a firm but not harsh end-feel.

If this is taken to its absolute limit, the *anatomical barrier* is engaged and this has a hard end-feel, beyond which any movement would produce damage.

If there is, for any reason, a restriction in the range of motion then a *pathological barrier* would be apparent on active or passive movement in that direction.

If the reason for the restriction involved inter-osseous changes (arthritis for example) the end-feel would be sudden, or 'hard'. However, if the restriction involved soft tissue dysfunction the end-feel would have a softer nature.

Kaltenborn summarizes end-feel variations thus:

- Normal soft end-feel is due to soft tissue approximation (such as in knee flexion) or soft tissue stretching (as in ankle dorsi-flexion).
- Normal firm end-feel results from capsular or ligamentous stretching (internal rotation of the femur for example).
- Normal hard end-feel occurs when bone meets bone as in elbow extension.

However pathological end-feel can involve a number of variations such as:

- A firmer, less elastic feel when scar tissue restricts movement or when shortened connective tissue exists.
- An elastic, less soft end-feel when increased muscle tonus restricts movement.
- An *empty* end-feel is one in which the patient stops the

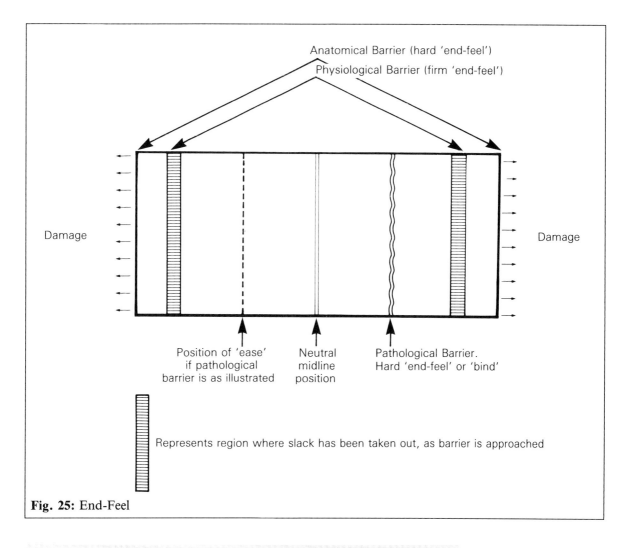

Anatomical Barrier (hard 'end-feel')

Physiological Barrier (firm 'end-feel')

Damage

Damage

Position of 'ease' if pathological barrier is as illustrated

Neutral midline position

Pathological Barrier. Hard 'end-feel' or 'bind'

Represents region where slack has been taken out, as barrier is approached

Fig. 25: End-Feel

movement (or asks for it to be stopped) before a true end-feel is reached, as a result of extreme pain (fracture or active inflammation) or psychogenic factors.

One objective of palpation of such restrictions is to establish the degree of limitation by establishing the range of motion in various directions. Another is the assessing of the nature of those restrictions through, among other factors (see p. 151) determination of the softness or hardness of the end-feel. Some manipulative techniques involve engaging the pathological barrier before a variety of methods are employed to increase the range of motion; pushing the barrier back, so to speak.

This can involve the use of isometric contractions of the agonist (shortened muscle or group of muscles) of their antagonists, as in Muscle Energy Technique, or it might involve active adjustment/manipulation as in chiropractic or osteopathic treatment. It might also involve mobilization using long leverage or use of joint play techniques. A different approach would be to move towards the direction opposite the direction of restriction, going away from the barrier, as in functional osteopathic techniques such as strain/counterstrain.

Whichever approach is used there remains the importance of knowing how to 'feel' the end of range of motion in any direction, without provoking sensitive tissues further. Practising on normal tissues and joints makes recognition of restricted ones simpler.

Kaltenborn states, 'The ability to see and feel the quality of movement is of special significance in manual therapy, as slight alterations from the normal may often be the only clue to a correct diagnosis.' If pain occurs anywhere in a range of movement (active or passive) which is preceded and followed by pain-free motion, the range in which the pain is noted is called a *painful arc*. Deviations of normal pathways during such a painful arc indicate avoidance strategies and are important diagnostically. As a rule *active movements* test all anatomical structures as well as the psychological willingness of the patient to move the area. *Passive movements* test only non-contractile tissues with such movements being compared with accepted norms as well as the corresponding opposite joint. End-feel, painful arcs, shortened muscles, restricted or exaggerated joint function, are all assessed this way. As a general rule a greater degree of motion is achieved passively than actively.

Chapter 7

Palpation of Joints and Functional Techniques and Palpation

The assessment of function of joints has been exhaustively covered in many osteopathic, orthopaedic and chiropractic textbooks over the past half century or more. The intent in this chapter is not to reduplicate such information but rather to summarize some of the most important elements of joint palpation, together with the provision of guides as to what some 'normal' ranges of motion might be expected to be. In addition some novel, sequential, approaches will be covered. Any serious student of joint palpation will need to seek elsewhere for more comprehensive descriptions.

Dysfunction of joints can be shown in three different ways, all of which form part of a comprehensive assessment of the musculoskeletal system: *observation, palpation and testing of function* (which is itself separated into active and passive movements).

We have already seen (Chapters 4 and 5) that there exist useful sequential screening patterns for uncovering evidence of shortened muscles (postural muscle screening) or changes within those muscles (NMT assessment, Nimmo's method etc). Mitchell, Moran and Pruzo, in their comprehensive text *An Evaluation of Osteopathic Muscle Energy Procedures* provide further useful guidance for practitioners wishing to find succinct methods for eliciting information as to where to focus attention, or where more detailed examination is required.

Such an approach is necessary since it is patently impossible during any normal consultation examination to cover each and every muscle, joint and test. As Mitchell puts it, 'The purpose... is to identify a body region, or body regions, which deserve(s) more detailed evaluation.' The following process of evaluation contains elements of the methods suggested by Mitchell, Moran and Pruzo, with many other researcher's ideas also being incorporated.

Each of the segments numbered below can be considered to be an individual exercise for anyone practising palpatory/observational skills, necessary for enhancing their ability to evaluate the mechanical and functional integrity of the musculoskeletal system. As expertise is gained in each individual segment the sequence could be combined with others, so that it becomes a more comprehensive evaluation exercise.

Note: Not all joints, or functions are covered. This book is not meant to provide detailed methods for structural and functional analysis, but rather to enhance the skills needed to do so.

Exercise 1. Observe the patient walking, slowly and briskly. Look for equal length of stride; good weight transfer from heel to lateral foot to metatarsal joints, with a push off from the big toe; external or internal rotation of legs; normal flexion and extension of hips, knees and ankles.

Pay particular attention to the presence or otherwise of a well developed arch during mid-stride on the weight bearing foot.

Normal gait should involve weight being placed evenly on each foot. Pelvis should remain virtually horizontal, with a slight sway being normal (more so in women). Observed from behind the spinal column curves from side to side, in a wave-like manner, with the greatest range in the mid-lumbar area. The thoraco-lumbar junction should remain above the sacrum at all times (also see notes on long leg/short leg later in this chapter).

Arm swing should come from the shoulder with little head motion. The upper shoulder fixators should appear relaxed. Look for asymmetrical patterns, stiffness and any tendency to rock or limp. Lewit also suggests 'listening' to the sounds made as the patient walks. In addition Lewit points out, 'Certain faults become more marked if the patient closes her eyes, walks on tiptoe or on the heels, and these should be examined as required.'

Always ask patients to adopt their typical work posture/position as part of the evaluation. Record all findings.

Exercise 2. Posture is then viewed from behind, attention being given to head balance (are ear lobes at the same height?); neck and shoulder symmetry, levels of scapulae, any lateral spine curves; the distance the arms hang from the side of the body, and folds at waist level (are they symmetrical?) gluteal folds (are they the same height from the floor?).

Side view is examined for normality of spinal curves; head position in relation to body; abdominal ptosis; winging of scapulae; angle of pelvic tilt; presence of foot arches; the way weight is distributed on feet. Record all findings.

Exercise 3. The patient stands facing the practitioner and symmetry of stance (foot placement) patella height, intercostal angle and clavicles are observed and recorded.

Side view is then evaluated. Is the head/centre of gravity over the body, or forward or backwards of it?

Patient is asked to bend backwards. Range should be around 35° with a sharp bend at the lumbosacral junction or at the thoracolumbar junction (in cases of increased mobility).

Antiflexion has a normal range of around 60° when knees are extended. Hamstring shortness affects this test, thus seated anteflexion is a more accurate assessment of lumbar flexibility.

Side-bending, with strict care that no ante- or retroflexion accompanies this, should achieve a range of 20° to each side. Assessment of range can involve (sighting from behind) evaluation of the shift achieved by the axilla, on the side away from which the patient is bending, as it comes to the end of the range of side-bending. This can be as far as being above a point beyond the lateral aspect of the buttock on the side to which the bend is taking place, or more normally to being above that buttock. A restricted excursion would be to a point above the intergluteal line (midline).

Hypermobility of the lumbar spine is, according to Lewit, indicated most strongly by hyperlordosis when standing relaxed together with exaggerated lumbar kyphosis when sitting relaxed.

Record all findings.

Exercise 4. The barefoot patient stands erect with back to squatting practitioner (eyes at level of iliac crests), patient's feet are apart, ankles directly below hip sockets (heels 4 to 6 inches apart), toes point straight ahead. Practitioner's hands are placed laterally inferior to iliac crests and are pushed in a superior-medial direction until the index fingers lie superior to the crest.

If heights of fingers from the floor are the same there is no anatomical leg length difference. If there is a difference (and there is no iliac rotation or spinal scoliosis) then an antatomical leg length difference can be assumed (see also later in this chapter the detailed segment on leg length discrepancy).

A slim book can then be used to equalize leg length until symmetry is achieved so that the following tests can be performed.

Is there an anatomical leg length difference? Can you balance iliac crest heights by 'building up' the short leg?

Exercise 5. Assessment of posterior superior iliac spine (PSIS) position is achieved by palpating on or just below the sacral dimples for osseous prominences. These are palpated for symmetry.

a. Is one anterior or posterior in relation to the other?

If one PSIS is anterior to the other then either the external rotators on that side (iliopsoas, quadratus femoris, gemellus (superior and inferior) and obturator (internal and external, if the hip is not flexed; piriformis if the hip is flexed), or the internal rotators on the other side, are short (gluteus medius and minimus and hamstrings, if the hip is not flexed, and adductor magnus and hamstrings, if it is flexed).

Posterior displacement indicates precisely the opposite pattern of shortening.

b. Is one PSIS superior or inferior to the other as you palpate?

Inferior displacement may involve short hamstrings, iliac or pubic dysfunction.

At this stage simply record whether one PSIS is anterior or posterior in relation to the other, and whether either PSIS appears superior or inferior, compared with the other.

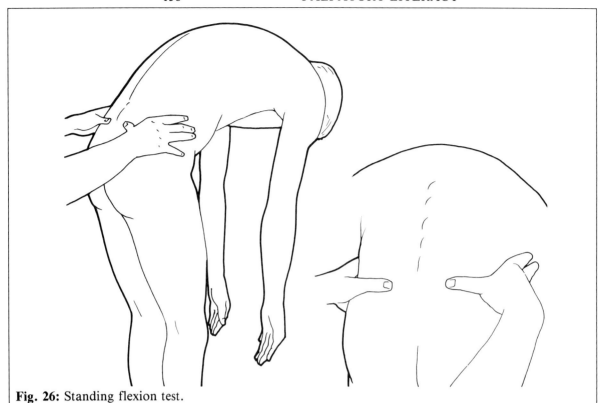

Fig. 26: Standing flexion test.

a) Palpate inferior slope PSIS. b) Patient forward-bends without bending knees.

Exercise 6. Standing flexion test; with thumbs placed firmly on the inferior slopes of PSIS, patient should be standing as in 4 above (iliac crests having been levelled by placing a slim book under the 'short' leg if asymmetry was discovered).

The patient keeps knees extended as he/she bends forwards to touch toes, your contact thumbs retain their positions on the same tissues overlying the PSIS. Assess the thumb which makes the greatest excursion as the patient bends fowards. Any additional movement of either thumb (PSIS) takes place due to the ilium being 'fixed' to the sacrum during final stages of flexion, indicating dysfunction (restriction) on that side. If hamstring shortness is responsible then this asymmetrical movement will not be seen when the same test is performed with the patient seated (described in Exercise 8, below).

The standing flexion test indicates ilio-sacral motion, since the muscular effort from the lower extremity is able to move the ilia in relation to the sacrum. This ability disappears when the patient is seated (see below) at which time the same test indicates sacral dysfunction (if asymmetry of PSIS movement occurs on flexion).

Did your thumbs move symmetrically? If not, which side is 'in lesion'?

Exercise 7. While the patient stands fully flexed the practitioner moves to a position so that the spine may be viewed from directly in front of the patient, for paravertebral (erector spinae) symmetry, or for evidence of greater 'fullness' on one side. Note what is found for comparison with subsequent evidence noted when the patient is seated (Exercise 9). Compare also with your findings from tests for tight postural muscles (Chapter 4) relating to quadratus lumborum and iliopsoas; repeat these now if necessary.

Mitchell suggests that if there is paravertebral fullness this is evidence of a degree of rotoscoliosis, and that if this is more evident in standing flexion than seated flexion, leg muscle tightness is probably a primary factor with the rotoscoliosis a compensatory feature.

If, however, seated flexion displays greater paraspinal fullness then rotoscoliosis is probably primary, with pelvic imbalance being compensatory.

If the evidence of fullness is the same seated and standing then rotoscoliosis is primary with no leg muscle compensation.

Is there increased 'fullness' in the paraspinal muscles? If so what does it relate to, according to Mitchell's guidelines, described above?

Exercise 8. Seated flexion test; evaluates sacro-iliac dysfunction and adds to evidence relating to erector spinae tightness.

Patient is seated on a low, firm surface, legs wide apart, hands

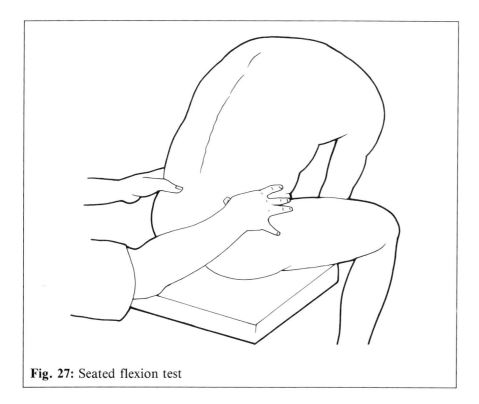

Fig. 27: Seated flexion test

behind neck. Practitioner is behind patient, eyes at level of PSIS. Thumbs palpate inferior aspect of PSIS, on both sides. The patient goes into a slow forward bend, as far as possible.

In this position the ischia are locked, making any motion between sacrum and ilia dependent on sacral freedom. This therefore helps to isolate sacro-iliac dysfunction.

The thumbs should be 'dragged' upwards to an equal degree if there is no restriction. If one thumb (PSIS) travels more superiorly than the other it indicates that there is a restriction of the sacro-iliac articulation, on that side. Further tests (not described here) are needed to determine whether torsion or flexion of the sacrum are involved.

Did the PSIS (and your thumb) move more on one side than the other?

Is there a sacro-iliac lesion, and if so, on which side?

Exercise 9. In this same position the fullness of the paravertebral muscles are observed by the practitioner moving to the front of the patient, and findings being interpreted as described in 7 above (rotoscoliosis and so on). If fullness is more apparent on one side during seated flexion, and there is no appreciable degree of rotoscoliosis, suspect quadratus lumborum shortening on this side. This can produce pelvic tilt as well as interfering with respiration (through influence on 12th rib or diaphragm).

Direct palpation of the lateral border of quadratus can give evidence of spasm or asymmetrical tightness, or a trigger point activity above the iliac crest.

Is their asymmetry in the paraspinal muscles during this test?

If so how do you interpet it?

Exercise 10. It is important in evaluating the evidence from the tests described so far that comparison be made with evidence of postural muscle tightness, as described in Chapter 4. Mitchell insists that, in addition, muscle weakness be examined and treated before conclusions are made as to pelvic (iliac or sacral) dysfunction. He gives the example of unilateral hamstring tightness preventing iliac motion and presenting a false positive test result, or a bilateral hamstring tightness preventing a true assessment of PSIS excursion from taking place, resulting in false negative findings in tests as described.

Therefore, at this stage, all muscles relating to pelvic function should be tested for length (and says Mitchell, strength) as described in Chapter 4. Is their hamstring short? On one or both sides?

What do tests for shortness of piriformis, tensor fascia lata and psoas show?

Exercise 11. You should also perform the F-AB-ER-E test, so called because it simultaneously assesses flexion-abduction-external rotation-extension, of the hip, in that sequence.

This test pinpoints hip pathology but also adds information which might be useful in pelvic dysfunction. Patient lies supine, practitioner stands on side of table closest to leg being tested. Patient flexes hip, allowing external rotation so that the foot of that leg rests just above the opposite knee. The knee on the tested leg is allowed to drop towards the table. It should reach a position where the lower leg is horizontal with the table. If this is not possible, carefully try to take it to that position by depressing the knee towards the floor.

Compare the range with the other side. If there is pain in the hip as the knee drops (or is taken) towards the floor, there is probably hip pathology.

Is there any hip dysfunction, evidenced by this test in your patient (model)?

Exercise 12. Mitchell and his colleagues also suggest other assessment be made of this region, such as the test for pubic tubercle height. This involves palpating the superior pubic crest (resting on the tubercles) with two index fingers. Deep palpation of the bony prominence of the tubercles allows assessment as to whether one is higher than the other.

If they are level there is no problem.

If one is higher it is only possible to discover which side is in lesion by referring to the standing flexion test (6 above). The side of lesion is shown by relative motion of the palpated PSIS in that test.

Does one side of the pubis palpate as being higher than the other?

If so, is that side superior or the other inferior?

You must refer back to the standing flexion test. If that showed an ilio-sacral lesion on one side, then that side of the pubis is the side that is dysfunctional.

Exercise 13. Ischial tuberosity height. The practitioner places the heels of his/her hands over the ischial tuberosities of the prone patient, with contact from the inferior gluteal folds directed towards the head. The most inferior aspect of the tuberosities is located with the thumbs and the relative height is assessed with eyes directly above them.

If they are level there is no lesion. If one is higher than the other it may usually be presumed to involve a superior subluxation on that side. This is confirmed by assessment of the sacro-tuberous ligaments. To test this the thumbs now slide in a medial and superior direction (towards the coccyx) bilaterally, until they meet the resistance of the sacro-tuberous ligament. If there is a superior ischium subluxation the ligament on that side will palpate as being slack compared with its pair.

Are the ischial tuberosities level?

If not which is superior?

Exercise 14. Apparent ('functional') short leg assessment. This is described in more detail later in this chapter. At this stage compare the levels of the internal malleoli, with the patient supine (where a short leg is likely to be due to iliosacral and pubic lesions) and prone (where a short leg is likely to be due to sacroiliac or lumbar lesions).

Is there an apparent short leg?

If so is this due to iliosacral or sacroiliac problems?

Exercise 15. Tests of ASIS positions indicate iliac rotation dysfunction and iliac flare patterns.

a. The patient lies supine and straight. Locate and palpate the inferior slopes of the anterior superior iliac spines (ASIS) with the thumbs and view from directly above the pelvis with dominant eye (see p. 15) in order to compare levels for superior/inferior asymmetry. If the ASIS are level there is no imbalance.

Now palpate to find the highest (nearest the ceiling) point of the ASIS bilaterally with the index fingers, and with dominant eye at midline of body and *eyes horizontal* with finger contacts, observe and compare for determination of which of these ASIS contacts is highest.

If one ASIS is more superior than the other it could indicate a posterior iliac lesion on that side, or an anterior iliac lesion on the other side. This is differentiated by comparison with results of standing flexion test (6 above).

For example if the flexion test revealed a left side iliosacral lesion, and the ASIS test showed left side superior this would indicate that there was a left side, posterior, iliac lesion.

Conversely if there was a right side lesion indicated by the flexion test, and a left side were superior in this ASIS assessment, it would indicate that this was due to a right anterior iliac lesion.

Spend a little time (draw a sketch, or examine the patient) working out why this is so if it appears confusing.

Is one ASIS more superior than the other?

If so does it relate to a posterior iliac lesion on that side, or to an anterior iliac lesion on the other side?

b. Now palpate, and place your thumbs on, the medial slopes of ASIS, with eyes above and directly over the midline. Compare the distances from the umbilicus (if scars make this unreliable use xyphoid as landmark instead) to ASIS contacts on both sides.

If the distances are equal there is no imbalance.

If there is a difference it could mean that on the greater side (longer distance from umbilicus to ASIS) an outflare of the ilium had occurred, or that an inflare had occurred on the shorter distance side.

Again reference to the standing flexion test gives the answer.

If the flexion test showed an iliac lesion on the right, and the ASIS-umbilicus distance is greater on that side, there is indeed an iliac outflare on that side.

What would it indicate if the flexion test (6 above) had shown an iliac lesion on the right, and the ASIS-umbilicus distance was greater on the other side?

What difference, if any, is there in the distances as you view them? What does it indicate in relation to your patient?

Exercise 16. Spinal assessment. Individual segments may be assessed for a variety of restrictions and motions; flexion, extension, side-bending (left and right), rotation (left and right) as well as such translatory movements as separation (traction), compression, and lateral and antero-posterior translations. These will be discussed in the context of 'functional analysis' later in this chapter.

General assessment is made by observing the patient standing, standing flexed, seated and seated flexed (knees straight and bent), as well as in such other positions (extension and so on) as may be desired by the examiner. The following exercises, *which are not meant to provide a completely comprehensive spinal assessment*, include methods derived from a number of texts, including:

- Osteopathic physician Sara Sutton's, 'An osteopathic method of history taking and physical examination' (*1977 Yearbook of Academy of Applied Osteopathy*, Colorado Springs).
- Karel Lewit's *Manipulation in Rehabilitation of the Motor System*, (Butterworth 1987).
- *Mobilisation of the Spine* by Gregory Grieve F.C.S.P.

Also much consulted in the devising of these exercises were the words of William Walton D.O. as set down in his excellent article 'Palpatory diagnosis of the osteopathic lesion' (*Journal of the American Osteopathic Association*, August 1971).

Exercise 17 a. Cervical spine palpation; with patient supine palpate posterior and anterior aspects of transverse processes for local tenderness.

In this position the pads of the middle fingers can be placed gently on the articular pillars of C2 to C7, successively, in order to palpate for any reduction in the symmetrical range of movement as the supporting palms of the hands take the head into forward and backward bending.

Also assess gross ranges of motion in rotation right and left, side-bending right and left as well as flexion and extension with patient seated. Place pads of thumb and third finger of one hand over the articular pillars of each vertebrae in turn (C2 to C7) while the other hand introduces the sequence of normal motions, successively.

With the head in full flexion the atlantoaxial joint may be palpated for restrictions in rotation. (Flexion locks joints below C2.)

For occiptoatlantal joint; patient supine, practitioner at head of the table. Patient is asked to first tilt head backward and then to tip the chin towards the chest. If the chin is observed to deviate to one side from the midline that is the side towards which the occiput is deviated.

What restrictions in normal motion did you find in this region using this approach?

b. Compare the results with the following, more precise palpation approach (Walton's).

The supine patient's head may be flat or on the flexed knee of the examiner, which is placed appropriately on the table. The occiput is cradled in the palms of both hands, leaving the pads of the fingers free to palpate the entire cervical spine, both lightly and deeply.

First the pads press lightly over the facets and transverse processes until palpable changes (tension, oedema, fibrosis, sensitivity, temperature changes, lessened skin elasticity and so on) are found. Increased pressure is then introduced to investigate for deeper changes in these tissues, such as oedema, deep muscular tension, interosseous changes and restrictions in mobility.

Flexion is assessed by placing the pads of the fingers between the spinous processes of the vertebral segments being palpated. The space is compared with that present in the more normal (i.e. no abnormal palpation signs) segments above or below.

Where an increased degree of separation is palpated check the segment by extending the head/neck at that level and assess the relative area of movement. If this is less than segments above and below then that segment can be stated to be 'locked in flexion'.

Similarly if the space between segments (between their spinous processes that is) palpates as narrower, compared with those above and/or below, this can be simply checked by introducing flexion and monitoring the degree/range of movement. If it seems less than it ought, as compared with its neighbours, it can be said to be 'locked in extension'.

Side-bending is assessed by placing the pads of the palpating fingers between the transverse processes while laterally flexing the cervical spine down to the segment being checked.

If this shows that transverse processes on one side (say left) are over-approximated, then side-bend to the right until the segment being checked should move (i.e. the transverse processes on the left should separate). If they fail to do so then that segment can be said to be 'lesioned', or 'subluxated', or 'locked', in side-bending to the left.

Rotation is assessed through use of deep palpation over the articular facets. If one feels more posterior than the one above or below it the cervical spine should be rotated towards the *opposite* side (away from the palpated posterior transverse process). If this fails adequately to rotate (compared with its neighbours) or even if it does rotate but with signs of increased tissue resistance, then it is said to be lesioned in rotation to the side of the posterior transverse process.

Usually this restriction will be to the same side as over approximated transverse processes (i.e. indicating a side-bending restriction) where there is a single segment lesion, or to the side of separated transverse processes, if a group side-bending lesion exists.

What findings did you make using this assessment as compared with the previous one?

Exercise 18 a. Thoracic palpation; patient seated, examiner places thumb on transverse processes of T1 to T3 successively as the patient first flexes, returns to neutral and then extends the head/neck repetitively, slowly, until evaluation is complete. Patient prone with chin on table, head in midline. Thumbs of examiner are placed sequentially on transverse processes of T4 to T9. Firm ventral pressure is exerted, after soft tissue slack has been removed, in order to evaluate rcsistance of each segment to hyperextension.

Rotation of the segment to the side of maximum resistance is assumed. The prone patient then arches the back by supporting the upper body on the elbows, chin on heels of hands. Practitioner is at head of table, palpating tips of transverse processes from T7 to L5 with thumbs, noting any increased posteriority, which indicates rotation to that side of the involved segment.

b. An alternative or additional evaluation could involve having the seated patient (straddling the table for stability is a good idea, or on a high fixed stool) in a variety of positions as follows.

With patient's arms folded, examiner stands at the side grasping further shoulder and fixing the other shoulder with his/her axilla. This leaves a hand free to palpate the tips of thoracic spinous processes for tenderness. Periosteal pain points on the spinous

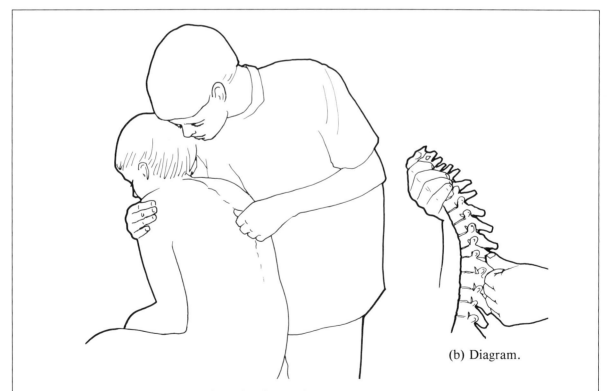

(b) Diagram.

Fig. 28: (a) Palpating tenderness of the tip of the spinous processes of the thoracic spine, separated by anteflexion.

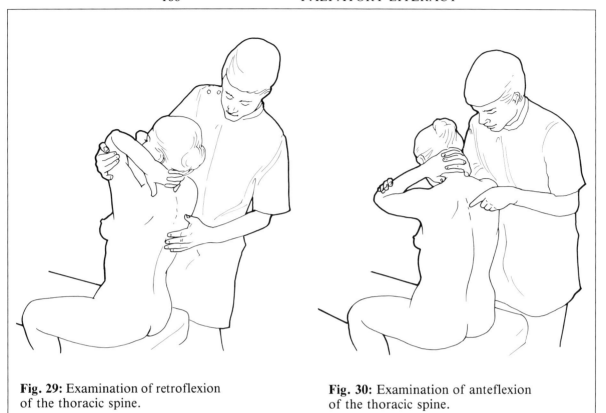

Fig. 29: Examination of retroflexion of the thoracic spine.

Fig. 30: Examination of anteflexion of the thoracic spine.

processes (see Chapter 4) indicate chronically increased tonus in the inserting muscles.

The patient then places hands behind neck, elbows together in front of the face. Both elbows are grasped in one of the examiner's hands, from below, allowing spinal extension to be easily introduced, as a finger of the other hand palpates between the spinous processes for the degree of movement and the end of the range of motion at each segment, sequentially. The patient is taken from neutral into retroflexion (backwards bending) and back to neutral, repetitively, slowly, until evaluation is complete.

The elbows are then held from above and sequential flexion is introduced as the tension of the end of the range of movement of each segment is assessed. The patient is taken from neutral into anteflexion (forward bending) and back to neutral, repetitively, slowly, until evaluation is complete.

For side-bending assessment the examiner stands behind the seated patient, one thumb resting on the interspace to be tested as the other hand introduces pressure towards the palpated side through the shoulder on the opposite side, to produce side-bending over the palpating digit. This palpating hand therefore acts as a fulcrum and the end range of motion is sequentially assessed in the thoracic spine.

Rotation is examined with the patient seated astride the table, hands behind neck. The examiner, standing to one side passes a hand across the chest to grasp the opposite shoulder, forearm lying across the chest. Flexion is introduced and the patient is sequentially rotated as the individual segments are palpated.

Rotation must be around the body's axis so that the palpating fingers (one each side of the spine) can palpate accurately the degree of rotation available in each direction.

What restrictions in normal motion did you find in this region using these methods?

c. Compare them with Walton's approach; after superficial stroking palpation of the seated patient's thoracic spine and paraspinal tissues any suspicious areas (evidenced by tension, tenderness, skin changes, oedema) are palpated more deeply, into the periaxial structures.

One side at a time is examined, with the operator standing to the side of the seated patient he/she wishes to assess. So if the right side of the thoracic spine were being examined the operator stands slightly behind and to the right of the patient. The operator's right hand is placed on the patient's left shoulder with the operator's forearm crossing behind the patient's neck, allowing the operator's elbow to rest on the patient's right shoulder. This gives the contact arm a great variety of possible directions of movement, controlling the patient into flexion, extension, side-bending and rotation with relative ease.

The free (in this case, left) hand is able to palpate any segment

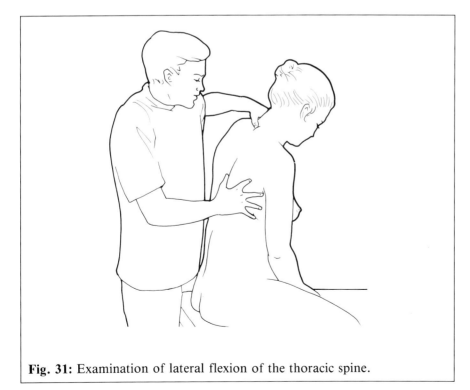

Fig. 31: Examination of lateral flexion of the thoracic spine.

(spinous process intervals and transverse processes as well as facet prominences) while motions are introduced by the right hand/arm. Obviously all hand positions (and the operator's position) are reversed for checking the opposite side.

After assessing the relative space between spinous processes, any which appear more widely separated than their neighbours are checked by the operator moving the contact arm to the front of the patient, grasping the opposite axilla, and introducing extension over the palpating thumb or finger(s). If the spinous processes fail to approximate when this is done then the superior one is probably locked in flexion.

With the control arm behind the patient's upper back again forced flexion is used to test the range of motion of any segments where over-approximated spinous processes have been palpated. Any which fail to flex adequately are locked in extension. Palpation with finger or thumb, between transverse processes identifies segments where approximation seems greater than in neighbouring segments. Side-bending is easily introduced (via the control hand or elbow) away from the palpating digit and if the transverse processes fail to separate then side-bending to that side is diagnosed.

Rotation is assessed by fixing, with a thumb pad, the transverse process and articular facet of the vertebrae below the one being checked. The control arm then introduces rotation up to the vertebra being tested. If it fails to move normally in rotation, say to the left, then it is said to be locked in rotation to the right. The articular facet of that vertebrae will be posterior on the side in which rotation is locked. Walton wisely warns that any restrictions in this area are possibly linked to viscerosomatic reflex activity producing paraspinal tension (see Chapter 4).

Exercise 19 a. Lumbar palpation; the patient is prone. This palpation involves sequential 'springing' of individual segments. It is performed with two fingers of one hand resting on the transverse processes of a segment, while the hypothenar eminence of the other, extended, arm rests over them. Slack is taken out and a springing movement to the floor is made as resistance is assessed. If resistance is palpated, and if there is pain, a restriction exists. If only pain is felt a disc lesion is possible.

With the patient side-lying these segments are again assessed, first with the patient anteflexed and then retroflexed.

What restrictions in normal motion did you find in this region so far?

b. Patient lies on side facing examiner, knees and hips are flexed. Examiner leans across patient while contacting bent knees with either his/her abdomen or thighs. Direct pressure is made through the long axis of the femurs which introduces retroflexion (backwards bending) to the lumbar spine.

The examiner's hands palpate individual segments, stabilizing with one hand the lumbar spinous process above the segment to be assessed, while a finger of the other hand lies between the spinous processes. After taking out the slack the segment is sprung by pressure through the femurs towards the palpating hands. On springing, a movement of the vertebrae below the one being fixed by the cephalid hand should be felt. If a 'blocked' segment exists then little or no motion will be palpated.

c. The patient lies on the side, knees and hips flexed, facing the examiner, who leans across the patient to fix (stabilize) the thoracic region with the cephalid forearm. The patient's knees and hips should be fully flexed so that their thighs press against their abdomen/chest, held there by the examiner's dorsal pressure to the lower legs, exerted by contact with his/her abdomen or thighs. This induces a great deal of anteflexion of the lumbar spine. The caudad forearm contacts the buttocks and repetitively increases and decreases anteflexion, as both hands palpate individual segments for decreased, increased, or normal ranges of flexion, as the region is gently sprung in this manner.

What restrictions in normal motion did you find in this region?

d. Walton suggests having the patient seated astride the end of the table with hands clasped behind the neck. The operator stands to the side and behind the patient, passing an arm through the 'loop' of the patient's arms on one side to rest the hand on the opposite upper arm. This provides control over flexion, extension, rotation and side-bending motions while the other hand palpates for normal mobility in the same manner as in thoracic examination described in 18c.

Exercise 20. The patient should be placed prone and the breathing 'wave' observed. This is a fan-like motion starting in the lumbar region and spreading to the upper thoracics when spinal mechanics are free. If there is restriction the movement will seem to stop.

Compare what is observed with findings of restriction during palpation (previous spinal assessment exercises) and the observed paraspinal 'fullness' in earlier assessments.

Exercise 21. Palpation for ribs locked in expiration (depressed ribs); palpation should be performed, from the side of table which brings the dominant eye over the centreline (see p.15). Examination is performed while the supine (knees-flexed) patient breathes deeply and steadily. The rib positions (right and left, same level) at full inhalation and exhalation are compared for relative rise and fall (upper ribs), as well as lateral excursion (lower ribs).

A digit resting on a rib which fails to rise (or move laterally) as far as its pair lies on a depressed rib, and there will usually be a series of these forming a group. It is necessary to identify the most cephalid of a group of ribs which fails to rise as far as its twin – this is the key rib locked in exhalation (i.e. it is depressed).

Just as such a rib can affect those below it so can one locked in inhalation (see below) affect those above it, making the most caudad of such a group the key one. 1st and 2nd ribs are often depressed, producing pain and numbness in the shoulder, suggesting thoracic outlet syndrome or scalene anticus syndrome, (anterior and medial scalene insert into first rib and posterior into 2nd). Such depressed ribs are often found in patients with asthma or obstructive pulmonary problems, or where there is a tendency to hyperventilation. If 1st and 2nd ribs are found to be depressed this calls for scalene involvement in a muscle energy manoeuvre.

If lower ribs are depressed then muscle energy methods which use the pectorals will assist in normalization. Tender points (see Chapter 5) for depressed ribs lie on the mid-axillary line (in the intercostal spaces).

What restrictions in normal motion did you find in this region?

Are there any depressed ribs?

Did you find a group of these, and if so did you identify the most cephalid of that group?

Do these findings correlate with tender points on the mid-axillary line at the same level?

Exercise 22. Palpation for elevated ribs; ribs restricted in inhalation are elevated. These are identified by palpation (one or two fingertips) in which the hands are placed flat on each side of the sternum, with wrists on the same plane as the hands (not flexed).

Maximum effort is called for in both inhalation and exhalation during testing. Motion of both bucket (up and down motion of upper ribs) and pump-handle (lateral and medial movement of lower ribs) movements is assessed. A palpating digit which is raised by the deep breathing, and which does not fall as far as its pair lies on an elevated rib. This is one which is locked in inhalation.

When an elevated rib is identified all pairs of ribs below are checked until a pair of normal ones are found (i.e. both rise and fall equally). The abnormal rib cephalid to the normal pair is the key rib (this being the most caudad of the elevated group) and probably affects all ribs above it. It is thus always essential to identify the most caudad of a group of elevated ribs.

The intercostals superior to an elevated rib will usually be sensitive and will palpate as tense. The fifth rib is commonly noted to be locked in elevation. There may be a deep radiating chest pain on deep breathing, and tightness in the pectoralis minor. Cardiac or pulmonary disease may need to be excluded. There may be swelling indicating costal chondritis. Treatment by muscle energy procedures is recommended.

Test all other ribs for range of motion and treat all those restricted. Tender points for elevated ribs lie at the angles of the ribs posteriorly. Rib interspace dysfunction tender points are found at the insertion at the sternum. These tender points often accompany over-approximated ribs.

What restrictions in normal motion did you find in this region?

Did you identify an elevated rib?

If so did you identify a group of these, and most importantly the most caudad of this group?

Did these findings correlate with tender points in the intercostal spaces around the angles of the ribs, posteriorly?

Did you palpate any interspace sensitivity, especially in the space above an elevated rib?

Exercise 23. Philip Greenman D.O. (*Principles of Manual Medicine*) suggests additional palpation processes for assessment of rib dysfunction. Sitting behind the patient, palpate the most posterior aspects of the rib cage from above downwards, feeling for a 'smooth' convexity which gets wider from above downwards. What is being felt for is any rib angle which seems to be more or less posterior than others. At the same time any increase in tone in the muscles overlaying or between the ribs (as well as pain) is sought. The muscles which attach to the angles of the ribs are the iliocostalis group and they become hypertonic when rib dysfunction occurs. Can you identify any rib dysfunction using this palpation?

Exercise 24. Palpate along the shafts of the ribs feeling for differences one from the other. The inferior margins of ribs are more easily palpated than the superior ones. Assess the intercostal width, evaluate differences in symmetry and feel for changes in tone in the intercostal muscles. Trigger points and fibrous changes may be found.

Move towards the spine and locate the articulation between the ribs and the transverse processes. Palpate these as the patient deeply inhales and exhales. Assess intercostal motion as well as rib mobility in relation to its spinal articulation.

Could you palpate all the elements described in this assessment?

Compare your findings with those established in your previous rib function assessments as outlined above.

Exercise 25. In Chapters 2 and 5 some of the exercises assessed elements of cranial and sacral rhythm function. The palpation exercise here is aimed specifically at learning more about cranial sutures and articulations. Whether or not you intend to use cranial osteopathic methods the exercise should be a useful one in enhancing your palpatory skills.

This exercise is performed on a living model/patient and in order to derive maximum benefit it is suggested that a good reference manual and a disarticulated skull be kept handy for reference and comparison of anatomical landmarks, suture patterns and general familiarization with individual articulations.

Extensive osteopathic research has shown that the sutures of the skull permit a degree of plasticity, or motion, and that the sutures themselves, in life, contain connective tissue fibres arranged in specific patterns related to the functional motions of the area. There are also blood vessels and small neural structures (including free nerve endings and unmyelinated fibres). The following palpation is not comprehensive as it leaves out most of the face and orbital structures. It is meant as a palpation exercise, not as a lesson in cranial work.

Start by having the supine patient lying without a pillow, yourself seated at the head of the table, forearms supported on the table, as you palpate, with pads of fingers, the vertex of the skull, just over half way posteriorly, for the saggital suture. Trace its path and note its pattern of serration which is wider posteriorly and narrows anteriorly.

As you move along this suture, anteriorly, you will come to the depression or hollow known as the bregma, where the coronal suture meets the saggital suture.

Now, using one hand on each side (finger pads) palpate laterally from the bregma along the coronal suture until you reach the articulation between the frontal and parietal bones. Are the sutures symmetrical? As your finger pad reaches the end of the coronal suture it will palpate a slight prominence, after which it reaches the pterion, the meeting point of the temporal, sphenoid, parietal and frontal bones. Moving slightly more inferiorly you will palpate the tip of the greater wing of the sphenoid, a most important contact in cranial work.

Move back to the pterion to follow the articulation between the parietal bone and the temporal squama. This curves backwards over the ear (the temporal squama is bevelled on its interior surface to glide slightly over this articulation).

Following this very subtle articulation you will reach the asterion, another junction point, this time between the temporal, parietal and occipital bones. Pass from the asterion superiorly (medially) along the lambdoidal suture until you once again reach the midline. Here the lambdoidal suture meets the saggital suture at the L-shaped lambda.

Move back again to the asterion and palpate your way towards the mastoid process along the occipital-mastoid suture, which will vanish below soft tissue as you approach the neck.

Never use more than a few ounces of pressure on these sutures when palpating. The time needed to do this palpation exercise well is at least 15 minutes. Repeat it many times, until these landmarks are familiar to you.

Functional Palpation of the Spine

Later in this chapter a series of exercises are given relating to assessments for short leg/long leg problems. As before this is not supposed to be totally comprehensive. It is a focusing exercise, bringing together aspects of what has been developed so far in the various palpatory and observational methods previously explained.

The following series of exercises includes reference to, and thoughts derived from, the research work of William Johnston D.O. (*Segmental*

Definition Part I and Part II *Journal of the American Osteopathic Association*, January 1988 and February 1988). Philip Greenman D.O. Professor of Biomechanics at the College of Osteopathic Medicine, Michigan State University (*Principles of Manual Medicine*) as well as descriptive observations from British osteopath Laurie Hartman D.O. (author of *Handbook of Osteopathic Technique*). Also included, later in this section (Exercise 31) is a functional exercise based on the work of the developer of Functional Technique, H.V. Hoover, D.O. ('A method for teaching functional technique' *1969 Yearbook Academy of Applied Osteopathy*).

Hartman analyses this 'indirect technique' saying that the operator's objective is to palpate the affected tissues, seeking 'for a state of ease and release, rather than looking for the point of bind and barrier', which characterizes so many other manipulative approaches (high velocity thrust, articulation, muscle energy methods and so on).

In the first instance an area (of the spine for example) is identified as being different, or abnormal as compared with the rest of the spine. The identification of areas of muscle fullness during the seated and standing spinal flexion tests (see pp.158ff.), or of 'flat' spinal areas, as described in the assessment sequence for tight muscles in Chapter 4, could direct you to such a 'different' area, requiring normalization. Hartman suggests another possibility, after initial suspicion has been alerted: 'Diagnosis of textural abnormality in the tissues is made in the normal way with palpation. A gradient of abnormality can be felt in a particular area and the centre of this area is made a focus.'

Hartman suggests light tapping be introduced over the spinous processes and paravertebral musculature to emphasize and localize the area of 'difference'. There will be a difference in the resonance noted which, he suggests, will be subjectively picked up by the patient, and which guides you to the most central portion of the dysfunctional tissues.

Exercise 26. Palpate the spine of a patient/model, assessing areas of flatness or fullness as you observe the flexed spine from the side or in front. Palpate the area and seek out the central site of tissue dysfunction, greatest hypertonia or sensitivity. Using the flexed fingertips of one hand tap lightly and steadily on the tissues identified as well as on those surrounding the area. Can you identify a different sound in the most affected tissues?

Once this has been identified, one hand (the 'listening' hand) is placed on the tissues; patient can be sitting, lying or standing. The other hand is used to introduce motion into the region, passively or with some active cooperation if directed to do so by the operator.

A sequence of motions is introduced to the region and in each instance (direction) the palpating hand, on the tense dysfunctional tissues, is feeling for greater ease or greater bind, trying to find a point where all the greatest points of ease (as assessed in all directions of motion - see below) are summated in order to achieve absolute

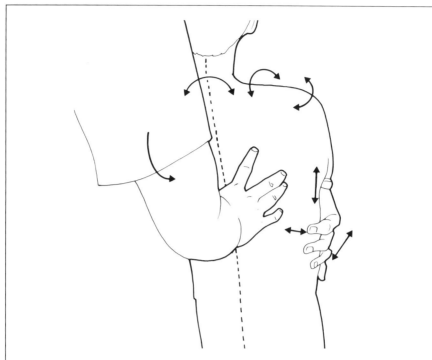

Fig. 32: Arrows show directions of movement as 'ease' and 'bind' are assessed by the 'listening' hand on the spinal tissues.
Movements are:
flexion-extension
rotation left and right
side-bending left and right
translation to each side
translation forward and back
translation up and down (traction and compression).

relaxation of the tissues. This, says Hartman, is a form of inhibition for the tense tissues, 'in that areas of irritability are quieted, the operator constantly looking for the state of ease and release'.

The movements introduced for assessment of ease and bind are:

- Flexion and extension
- Side-bending both ways
- Rotation both ways
- Translation anterior and posterior
- Translation laterally, both ways
- Translation cephalic and caudad (traction and compression)
- Followed by respiration involving both inhalation and exhalation.

Greenman describes the process of achieving the sequentially arrived at point of ease if the first six motions as 'stacking' (the order in which these are applied is not significant incidentally; simply it is useful to apply them sequentially so that none are forgotten). This must however be followed by the final respiratory screening for maximum ease.

The timing of each stage of respiration can be anywhere from 5 to 30 seconds. A new balance point is sought in each of the various motion directions as the respiratory effort is repeated, until restrictions are released, and mobility improved. A sense of a wider range of normal (greater ease) should be felt by the operator as these releases occur.

Exercise 27. Greenman describes a sequence of exercises for achievement of 'functional literacy'. The following is a modified summary of his sequence. Stand behind and to the side of a seated patient/model whose arms are folded, so that their hands are holding their opposite shoulders. Place a 'listening' hand somewhere on the upper thoracic spine where tissue tightness, fullness, have been identified. Allow the hand to be very still. Wait until it feels 'nothing' (no movement). The other hand ('motor' hand) should be placed on the patient's head, which it leads through specific motions such as flexion and extension (very slowly performed, without jerking).

The palpating hand tries to identify tissue changes in terms of increased ease or increased bind. Keep repeating flexion, back to neutral, flexion, back to neutral, noting where the point of maximum ease is. Then introduce slow repetitive backward bending of the head as you palpate for ease. Is the ease greater with the head flexed or extended?

Return to neutral and introduce side-bending right and rotation to the left, of the head and neck on the trunk, several times (back to neutral after each excursion) and then side-bending left and rotation to the right of the neck and head on the trunk, all the while palpating the dysfunctional area for alterations in ease or bind characteristics. Do the tissues relax or become more tense?

Find the point – somewhere between extreme side-bending left-rotation right and side-bending right-rotation left – in which the palpated tissues feel at their most relaxed.

Is their symmetrical range of ease and bind to both sides?

Where in this combination movement is there the most ease in any given direction?

Go back to neutral and introduce, and try to combine, the following movements as you palpate for ease and bind: small amount of forward bending, accompanied by right side-bending and right rotation, of the head and neck on the trunk; follow this with slight flexion, side-bending left and rotation, of the head and neck on the trunk to the left.

Palpate constantly for ease in the thoracic segment under your listening hand. Evaluate the symmetry of the findings.

Was ease/bind found at the same place left and right?

Greenman suggests that similar palpation exercises be performed in

various regions of the spine. In each case what you are looking for in
normal tissue, or where there is only minimal dysfunction, is a wide
range of motion accompanied by minimal signalling (i.e. most of it is
in relative 'ease').

Where significant degrees of dysfunction exist there will be narrow
ranges of position which produce signals of ease or decreased bind.
Experience is the only teacher as to what is and what is not significant
clinically.

Johnson explains the terms direct and indirect as follows:

> When the incremental aspects of these cues [directions of motion
> restriction] are appreciated as an immediately increasing resistance
> towards a sense of barrier in one direction, and an immediate increasing
> ease towards a sense of potential release in the opposite direction, then
> the terms direct [towards the sense of resistance] and indirect [away from
> the sense of resistance] offer a classification of osteopathic manipulative
> procedures, based on diagnosed asymmetry, to be addressed.

It is easy to move from such a diagnostic assessment into active
treatment. His summary of the planning and criteria involved in a
functional approach to treatment can be expressed as follows:

a. It is necessary to introduce motion in any one direction at a time
which involves minimal force.
b. Motion direction is towards a sense of increasing ease which is
manifested by a lessening in the sense of resistance to pressure
from the palpating fingers.
c. Combinations of direction elements are combined, such as
rotation and translation, producing variations in torsion.
d. Active respiration is also monitored for its influence on 'ease'.
e. The examiner follows the continuous flow of information
signalling increasing ease/decreasing resistance during all
procedures.

Exercise 28. Patient is seated, operator stands behind and to one
side, *palpating a previously identified area of dysfunction in the
thoracic spine*. Adopt a contact where the patient has arms folded
and you embrace the shoulder furthest from you with one hand,
drawing the opposite shoulder into your axilla, so that you have the
ability to control the various directions of motion.

Sequentiallly introduce the elements of forward bending followed
by backward bending, left side-bending, right side-bending, rotation
left, rotation right, then a combination of side-bending in one
direction with rotation to that side during flexion and then extension.
Then introduce side-bending in the other direction with rotation to
the opposite side during flexion and then extension. Add to positions
of 'maximum ease' thus discovered elements such as translation
anterior and posterior, translation from side to side, and translation
cephalid and caudad, to the positions of maximum ease uncovered in
order to discover where the maximum point of ease occurs.

Can you sense ease and bind?

Can you find a 'most easy' position, by combining elements of these motions?

Exercise 29. Perform exactly the same sequence *on a segment lower down the spine which does not display evidence of dysfunction.* Compare your findings of range and position of ease and bind with the previous exercise.

Exercise 30 a. Repeat all the components of Exercise 27, but now introducing long-held (as long as is tolerable to the patient) breath, in both inhalation and exhalation, in those positions in which maximum ease was palpated. Is there any additional release (or increase) of resistance during or after either phases of held breath? The secret of this approach is learning to apply all specific directions of motion which enhance ease, along with the respiratory component which produces maximum ease.

b. Repeat the sequence of Exercise 27, but this time identify the most extreme positions of bind, so that you can eventually engage the restriction barrier (exactly the opposite from what you were doing in 27 and 29a). In this position (whatever combination of sequence has led to increased bind) have the patient gently try to return to the starting position (normal) against your resistance for a ten-second 'hold'.

Retest the area of resistance after this and see whether you have increased the range, pushed back the barrier, increased ease? This is a muscle energy procedure in which an isometric contraction of the tight soft tissues has allowed an increase in their elasticity after the contraction. Which approach appeals to you most, seeking ease, or obliging the barrier to retreat after engaging it?

The developer of functional technique, H.V. Hoover D.O., explained the essence of this approach in the words of the founder of osteopathy, Andrew Taylor Still. 'I am doing what the body tells me to do'. He asks the beginner to perform the following three 'experiments' which we are grouping together as Exercise 30. In each case a question is posed, the answer to each being 'yes'. The proving of the accuracy of those answers will tell you whether you are ready for this method – whether you have achieved palpatory literacy.

Exercise 31 a. Question 1: Does the clavicle move in a definite and predictable manner when demands are made upon it by definite movements of an adjacent part? Standing facing the seated patient place the pads of the (relaxed) fingers of your right hand, lightly over the right clavicle, just feeling the skin overlaying it. This hand is the 'listening' hand. It is there to listen to what happens.

With your left hand hold the right arm just below the elbow (this is your 'motor' or moving hand). The patient must be relaxed, passive and cooperative, not helping or hindering the introduction of movements by your hand. The feeling hand should barely touch the skin, no pressure at all being applied to the clavicle.

Raise and lower the arm slowly several times until you are certain that there is no shoulder movement, that you have the weight of the arm without assistance from the patient. Now the exercise proper begins.

Slowly take the arm backwards from the midline just far enough to sense a change in the tissues under the palpating hand. Do not move quickly or wiggle or jerk the arm, so that the sensations being felt by that hand are accurately perceived. Repeat this several times, slowly, so that you become aware of the effect of a single, simple, movement (remember the question you have been asked).

Now take the arm forward of the midline and again assess the effect on the palpated tissues (clavicle and surrounding tissue). Abduct and then adduct the arm, rotate the arm outwards and subsequently inwards, each time slowly and if necessary repeatedly, noting the tissue response to that single direction of movement.

What response was noted to single physiological movements?

b. Question 2: Are there differences in ease of motion and feeling of tissues of this clavicle when it is caused to move in different physiological motions? Follow the same starting procedure until the exercise proper begins. Move the patient's arm backwards into extension very slowly as you palpate the changes in the tissues around the clavicle. Compare the feeling of the tissues as you take the arm into flexion, bringing it forwards. Now compare the feelings in the receiving hand as you abduct and then adduct the arm, slowly, deliberately, gently.

Compare the tissue changes as you first internally and then externally rotate the arm.

Did there appear to be directions of motion which produced altered feelings of 'ease' in the tissues?

c. Question 3: Can the differences of ease of motion and tissue texture be altered by moving the clavicle in certain ways?

Repeat the introductory steps up until the exercise proper begins. Flex the patient's arm, bringing it forward of the midline, slowly and gently until you note the clavicle moving or the tissue texture under the palpating hand changing. Stop at that point.

Now extend the arm backwards from the midline, slowly and gently until you note the clavicle moving or the tissue texture under the palpating hand changing. Stop at that point. Find a balance between these two states, a point of balance from which movement in any direction causes the clavicle to move along with a change in tissue texture. Hold this point of physiological balance, which Hoover calls neutral.

Starting from this balanced point you should next find the point of balance between adduction and abduction. Again starting from the point of balance (between flexion and extension as well as adduction and abduction) you move on to find the point of balance between internal and external rotation. You have now achieved a state of reciprocal balance between the arm and the clavicle. From here Hoover leads you to another important finding.

d. With the arm and clavicle in reciprocal balance, as at the end of (c) above, see whether you can move through the six physiological motions to see which of these, singly, gives a sensation of improving tissue texture compared with the other physiological motions. One of the directions may be found which does not increase 'bind', or increases 'ease', more than the others.

Having found this motion, slowly and gently continue to repeat it for as long as the sensory hand continues to report that tissue conditions, motion of the clavicle, are gaining in 'ease'. Should bind begin to be noted as this is done, Hoover suggests that the various directions of motion are rechecked, to find that which introduces the most ease. If none do then stop at this point, noting what it is that you have been feeling. If a further direction of motion producing ease is found, this is repeated until bind seems to occur again. Repeat the retesting procedure of various directions of motion.

Hoover says:

> This process of finding the easy physiological motion and following it until bind starts and then rechecking may go on through two or more processes until a state of equilibrium is found from which tissue texture indicates ease *in all physiological motion.*

e. In order to perform this final part of Hoover's experiment the untreated, opposite clavicle should be taken through stages (a), (b) and (c). At this point, having reached a reciprocal balance between arm and clavicle, reliance is placed on the tissues to 'tell' you what movements are required by it to achieve maximum ease:

> The operator relaxes and becomes entirely passive as his sensory or listening hand detects any change in the clavicle and its surrounding tissues. A change in the clavicle and its surrounding tissues, if felt, by the sensory hand, sends the information to the reflex centres which relay an order to the motor hand to move the arm in a manner so as to maintain the reciprocal balance, or neutral. If this is the proper move there will be a feeling of increasing ease of motion and improved tissue texture. This process continues through one or more motions until the state of maximum ease or quiet is attained.

This is of course very much the objective Upledger seeks in fascial unwinding methods as discussed in Chapter 5. This method can be employed, with the addition of translation motions, for any extremity or spinal joint, as a means of identifying directions of ease and bind. The choice then remains yours, whether to use functional or active approaches in restoring normality (as in the two methods described in Exercise 30).

Notes on Palpation and Evaluation of Long Leg/Short Leg Problems   **An Exercise in**
The following notes and exercises relate to an all-too common   **Palpatory Literacy**

musculoskeletal problem, and are meant to help the reader to integrate their palpatory and assessment skills. *These notes should not be considered to be definitive on this topic, although they do include the opinions and methods of many leading clinicians. They provide a starting point for using palpatory skills in a complex setting for those who wish to explore body mechanics.*

The major usefulness of this section will be to encourage the use of palpatory skills to both joint and soft tissues through the use of the exercises. Before coming to these exercises it may be necessary to explain the viewpoints of a number of experts (some of whom disagree on aspects of the problem) so that what is being palpated and evaluated makes some sense. Refer also to the pelvic and spinal assessments, discussed in this chapter.

Mitchell, Moran and Pruzo, who were extensively referred to earlier in this chapter, make the following observation regarding 'functional', or apparent, short leg assessment. They stress that the assessment is needed to give evidence of the success or otherwise of subsequent treatment, offering a 'baseline' from which to work.

The height of the pelvic (iliac) crest as assessed with the patient standing (see Exercise 4, this chapter) gives evidence of an anatomical leg length difference. To assess for a functional (apparent) short leg the patient is first placed supine, lying quite straight. The distances of the inferior slopes of the internal malleoli, from the trunk, are compared by placing the thumbs on them and the eyes directly over them.

If one side is higher there is an iliosacral lesion on that side producing this apparent shortness (presuming the iliac crests were level when the patient was standing). Retest for an iliosacral lesion with the patient performing the standing flexion test as PSIS excursion is noted.

If no shortness is observed, with the patient supine place the patient in a prone position, lying straight. Again measure and compare by viewing medial malleoli, with the thumbs on their inferior slopes.

If the malleoli are level there is no functional shortness. If one is shorter (i.e. the malleolus is closer to the trunk) it is on the side of a sacroiliac lesion. Retest for a sacroiliac lesion by performing the seated flexion test with thumbs on the PSIS, looking for the one which has the greatest excursion on flexion of the patient.

A variety of iliosacral, sacroiliac, pubic and lumbar lesions may cause this apparent shortness according to Mitchell, Moran and Pruzo. Fryett (*Principles of Osteopathic Technic*) says:

1. Legs are usually of unequal length, running to as high as 90 per cent of people.

2. This is probably a major cause of sacroiliac dysfunction.

3. Other factors such as:
   - unilateral psoitis
   - unequal lumbar tension
   - shortened fascia in the hip region
   - shortened or relaxed ligaments
   - flat feet

may all make the legs appear to be of unequal length when actually they are not.

4. Measuring to identify short-leg problems is best achieved by X-ray. To avoid distortion the tube must be absolutely in the centre of the target, horizontal to the heads of the femur, patient standing still, knees extended. This gives accurate definition of the height of the trochanters (to within $\frac{1}{4}$ of an inch) but distorts the sacrum and lumbar spine.

5. All individuals with leg length differences (no matter how slight) have a degree of functional disturbance of the S/I joints, unless a heel-lift correction has been made.

6. Bone, young and old, is plastic, and conforms with Wolff's Law which states, 'Every change in the use or static relations of a bone leads not only to a change in its internal structure and architecture but also to a change in its external form and function.'

7. In chronic cases the S/I joint is not perfectly normal in form and cannot be treated as though it were. As a rule the problem has been present since the patient first began to walk.

8. Compensation always occurs, sometimes adequately, so that severely lopsided, deformed pelves, associated with leg-length differences of up to half an inch, may produce no pain whatever.

9. Fryett does not like the term 'short' leg, for often the problem is one of a long leg. He points out that the degree of load carried by a leg will influence its growth. Some authorities believe that right-handed people brace themselves more on the left leg which develops more than does the right. Many right handed people have a left foot which is larger than their right in consequence. Janda has pointed out that we spend at least 80 per cent of our time standing on one leg (when we are not sitting or lying down that is).

10. The angle of the neck of the femur varies, normally being about 125°. If it inclines towards the perpendicular however (coxa valga) it would appear to make the leg longer than normal. The opposite situation, an inclination more to the horizontal (coxa vara) tends to make the leg shorter than normal.

11. The idea of increasing the length of a short leg is not futile, Fryett insists. It is always worth trying in the young. Where there is no apparent pathology in a child with unequal leg lengths, it is safe to assume that it is the short leg that is 'at fault'.

12. *Gray's Anatomy* instructs us that, 'Growth in leg length of the femur takes place chiefly from the lower epiphyses.' This is on line with the adductor tubercle.

Fryett's Treatment

He suggests attention to the epiphyses of the femur, tibia and fibula. All these receive attention from Fryett (he 'manipulates and tries to stretch' these epiphyses) in order to try to encourage greater circulation at the openings for the arterial supply to these bones. He also encourages hopping and kicking (a football for example) with the short leg, and adjusts the heels of young patients, while they are on a pair of scales, so that they carry more weight on the shorter leg.

Discussing the general effects of such anomalies Fryett reminds us that it may be necessary to deal with more than the local and obvious: 'There is a law in physics to the effect that stress in any mechanism will spread until it is absorbed, or until the mechanism breaks down.'

Physiological Assessment (Fryett)
1. If we have a normal or exaggerated A/P lumbar curve the bodies of the lumbar vertebrae rotate to the low side. If, for example, there is a long left leg, the right side of the pelvis will be low and if the A/P curve is normal the bodies rotate to the right. Treatment (according to Fryett) should involve lowering the left side in the hope of thus levelling the base plane and correcting compensatory lesions.
2. To the degree that the lumbar spine is in flexion the bodies are forced to rotate to the high side. Therefore if we find vertebrae rotated to the high pelvic side we know that, whatever the appearance, those vertebrae are abnormally posterior.

In such a case a heel lift is contraindicated. The best approach is to increase the A/P curve. As the curve passes into the normal range the vertebrae (the body, not the spinal process) will release and rotate to the low side.

This may require release of contracted, shortened psoas muscle(s), as this can hold the lumbar spine in exaggerated flexion (see below for more on psoas and other associated muscles).
3. If there are problems of restricted motion with the SI joint(s) or the lumbar vertebrae, then heel lifts are deferred until these problems have been dealt with by mobilization (adjustment, Muscle Energy methods, stretching exercises and so on).
4. Any leg length adjustment by means of heel-lifts in a chronic case should not exceed an eighth of an inch initially. This small change is often enough to allow compensation to take place. Too large a compensating lift can create excessive demands in terms of adaptation requirements and an increase in symptoms. 6 weeks later after reassessment a further lift may be used.
5. Fryett suggests that in some instances (and he does not know why) it is better to lower the long leg. This can be done by removing part of the heel of ALL shoes currently being worn.
6. In some instances all symptoms associated with poor compensation can be relieved by manipulative work without any lifts. This may be the best first approach, using methods which stretch all shortened postural muscles (see tests below and in Chapter 5).

Mennell (*Back Pain*) suggests that Achilles tendon tightness be assessed. In using lifts he says that store-bought shoes can never be raised at the heel by more than half an inch without throwing stress onto the foot as a whole, due to alteration of the slope of the sole. This can be overcome by raising the sole as well. When there is any shortness of the Achilles tendon a full correction of heel height must not be attempted or the remaining resilience in the tendon will be lost. He places great emphasis on identification and correction of TFL shortness related to low back and SI joint problems (see below and Chapter 5).

Cailliet (*Low Back Pain Syndrome*) says that measuring from the ASIS to the malleolus (as suggested by some experts) is at best inaccurate and offers little of significant value. He suggests three landmarks:

1. Standing barefoot both legs close together, fully extended at the knees. Examiner places fingers on pelvic brim and determines the horizontal levels of his fingertips. This is quite accurate.
2. Note the dimples over the SI joints (where the gluteus maximus attaches to the periosteum over the sacrum), and estimate from these the pelvic level. This will only be difficult when the patient is very overweight or underweight (see Exercises 6 and 8, above, for more on pelvic palpation/assessment).
3. Observe the lumbar spine at its 'takeoff' from the sacrum. The posterior-superior spines of the vertebrae are usually prominent and observable. If an oblique take-off is seen this implies obliquity of the sacral base.

If these three clinical methods indicate a leg-length discrepancy, the exact amount of this can be assessed by using a series of boards of varying thickness (1/8, 1/4, 1/2, 3/4 and 1 inch). These can be placed under the foot of the short leg until the pelvis reaches a balanced level.

Cailliet insists that it is, after all, a level pelvis (and therefore a straight spine) which we desire, rather than leg symmetry. He reminds us that a history of polio, or genu valgum or varum, or a previous fracture may all result in significant leg length discrepancies. It is only the effect on pelvic and spinal mechanics which matter.

Lewit (*Manipulative Therapy in Rehabilitation of the Motor System*) has much to say on the subject of short legs. He reminds us that an artificial difference of more than 1 centimetre (less than half an inch) in leg length, changes the balance in the coronal plane, and is immediately felt and resented, whereas raising both heels is hardly noticed. Using a plumb line Lewit observes for lateral shift of the pelvis from the mid-line.

Note: This can be used to test spinal mechanics in patients if we insert heelpads and watch the changes in deviation.

Reaction to unequal leg length (as presented by patient or initiated by operator) is normal if:

1. There occurs a convex curve to the low side.
2. There is rotation of the vertebral bodies to the low side (provided there is a lordosis, in agreement with Fryett).
3. The lumbo-dorsal junction remains vertically above the sacrum.
4. The pelvis as a whole shifts to the high side.

Note: If there is an obliquity of the sacral base on standing this should always be observed again on sitting. If it remains when seated then the cause is not a short leg. (We should therefore compare sitting and standing sacral obliquety before using Cailliet's boards.)

Testing for equal weight distribution requires standing on two scales and ensuring that they display more or less equal weights. Only then can a plumb-line assessment be valid. As heel lifts are placed for the assessment of deviation, the weight must be seen to be equally balanced. If weight is placed on one foot more than the other the whole body deviates to that side with the head deviating furthest.

The patient should be assessed for weight distribution on two scales, with and without a heel-pad on the lower side (of the pelvis). A subjective reaction should also be sought: do they feel happier with or without the pad? If there is a one-sided flat-foot, an arch support is likely to be more effective than a heel lift.

Lewit agrees that leg length is of no concern unless is causes obliquety at the sacral base and the spine. How to measure differences, he says, is beside the point, for what is important is what we see on X-ray in relation to spinal mechanics.

Pathological Findings Related to Short Leg (Lewit)
1. A tilt (obliquety) without compensating scoliosis, or with insufficient scoliosis, so that the lumbo-dorsal junction does not find itself above the lumbosacral juntion.
2. No pelvic shift to the high side.
3. No rotation of the vertebral bodies when there is a scoliosis and lordosis, or actual rotation to the opposite side from the scoliosis (away from the convexity), or scoliosis to the high instead of the low side.

Objectives of Correction Involving Heel Lifts
1. The achievement of a sufficient degree of compensation to bring the lumbodorsal junction over the lumbosacral junction (or close to this point).
2. A return of the pelvis from the high side to the centre.
3. A decrease in the degree of scoliosis.

In some instances of complex pelvic distortion a leg may appear shorter in the supine position, while on sitting this is reversed. There is usually a muscular 'blockage' involving spasm of the iliacus, and/or there may be imbalance between the gluteals.

Lewit suggests that an assessment should also always be made of any difference in leg length *below* the knee, by having the supine patient bend both knees, feet on the table. The knee which is highest in relation to the table belongs to the long leg.

Bailey and Beckwith (*Academy of Applied Osteopathy Yearbook 1966*) summarized their analysis of over 400 cases of short leg determined by standing X-ray. Average shortness was 0.88 cm, 53 per cent were left sided. In 88 per cent of short leg the iliac crest was low on the side of shortness. In 72 per cent the upper border of the sacrum was low on the short side. In 39 per cent the symphysis had deviated to the short side. It was in the midline in 30 per cent.

Strachan (*Academy of Applied Osteopathy Yearbook 1966*) says that lifts should be used with care in stiff spines. Age should not be the deciding factor but rather the mobility of the spine and therefore its ability to adapt to new demands. In children a lift almost equal to the difference in leg length is suggested. Lateroflexion mobility is important in deciding whether to use a lift. If restricted unnaturally this should be dealt with prior to a lift being used, if one is indicated.

Spinal distortions caused by short legs occur low in the spine. Lateral curves which do not include at least two lumbar vertebrae are unlikely to be helped by a lift, even if a short leg is present. A lift is most beneficial if there exists a low sacrum on that side and a lumbar side curve convex on the short side. Any variations on that simple picture may be complicated by lifts.

Williams (*Lumbosacral Spine*) tells us that a lift in such an instance is called for *unless* there is pain radiating into the short extremity. If pain is into the long extremity then a compensatory lift on the short side often relieves nerve pain. If there is nerve pain in a leg which seems to relate to foraminal encroachment, and there is no leg length difference, a temporary lift on the opposite extremity may relieve symptoms.

Exercise 32. Observe your patient's/partner's pelvic landmarks (pelvic brim, S/I 'dimple', spinal 'take-off' angle) and decide:

Palpation/Evaluation Exercises

a. Is there a short leg, and if so which side is it on?
b. Do the spinal and pelvic changes reflect good or poor adaptation to a short leg (see list under Exercise 34)?
c. Check for piriformis, psoas, TFL and Achilles tendon shortness, flat feet, as well as spinal mobility and side-bending limitations (ask yourself what these findings mean in relation to short leg problems).
d. If you have a plumb line assess lateral shift of body.

Exercise 33. Compare the pelvic/spinal changes standing and seated.
  Is the 'low' side still low?
  If not what does it mean?

Exercise 34. If there is no leg length discrepancy use a pad, folded paper or other tool to raise first one heel (increasing leg length) and then the other. In each case observe for normal or abnormal changes, bearing in mind the differences which occur when there is a normal or exaggerated lumbar curve and when this is flat.

a. Is the lumbar spine convex towards the low side (short leg)?
b. Do the vertebral bodies rotate towards that side?
c. Is there a pelvic shift to the high side?
d. Is the lumbodorsal junction directly over the lumbosacral junction?
Decide whether the spinal mechanics are normal or not.

Exercise 35. Assess all the findings from the above and decide whether or not a lift is required.

Does a lift produce the normalization which Lewit demands? Now go through De Jarnette's sequence and compare results with the above.

De Jarnette and the Short Leg

Much of SOT (sacrooccipital technique) work depends upon assessment of a short-leg and associated dysfunction. *Heel tension* is usually assessed since the achilles with the greatest tension is the strong leg (in most cases). The complexities of defining category 1, 2 and 3 patients in SOT, and the use of supporting blocks to normalize leg-length, together with a host of odd 'signs' (dollar sign, crest sign, fossa signs and so on) defy easy explanation, so this will not be attempted. If these concepts interest you try to learn SOT from professional seminars.

In a handbook of chiropractic first aid, De Jarnette provides the following insights into short leg problems:

Patient is supine, grasp ankles and pull these into extension and assess for the superior inner malleolus, thus identifying the short leg. Correct the long leg first by placing the foot of that leg on the extended knee of the short leg, rotating the hip externally so that the knee of the flexed (long) leg falls towards the floor. Hold this stretch until relaxation of the tense musculature is felt (half a minute or more). Go back to a normal supine position.

Next hold the ankle of the short leg firmly with one hand, having flexed that leg at the knee, and adduct the knee so that it is forced across the extended knee of the long leg. Pull the ankle laterally to increase stretch in the musculature around the pelvis/hip area, holding this position for 40 seconds (there may be some discomfort).

Patient lies with feet flat on table, knees flexed and well separated. Hold the knees in this position as patient tries strongly to bring them together for 10 seconds or so.

Same position but this time knees are together, as patient tries strongly to separate these while you resist for 10 seconds or so. The resisted approximation and separation are repeated alternately, 3 times each, in order to improve tone in the supporting soft tissues of the SI joints and pelvis.

This sequence is recommended by De Jarnette for low back, hip and leg problems of many types.

Exercise 36. Go through this entire De Jarnette sequence after you have performed all the assessments described above (Exercises 31–34) and then see whether a reassessment (after De Jarnette's sequence) gives you any different information or indications. Also incorporate elements from the suggestions in the following notes on specific muscle assessments.

Additional notes on palpation/assessment methods for specific muscles which can often be involved in short leg problems
(see also Chapter 4 for specific tests for shortness of these muscles).

Are TFL or Psoas Overactive?

Exercise 37. The side-lying patient has his/her pelvis firmly stabilized by the operator who simultaneously palpates the trochanter of the upper side (side being tested). The untested (lower) leg is slightly flexed at hip and knee. The tested leg is extended at the knee and slightly hyper-extended at the hip. The operator's whole hand is over ASIS also palpating the trochanter.

Abduction of the extended leg, actively, should take it through 45° against slight resistance from the operator's other hand. Movement must be felt in the trochanter (it slips away) if the leg, rather than the whole pelvis, is being moved. If performed normally this is graded as a 5 or 4 (Janda).

Lewit suggests that in this position the cephalid hand resting on the anterior pelvis should be placed so that the fingers rest on the TFL and the thumb on gluteus medius. The caudad hand is on the lower thigh applying resistance as the leg is abducted. In this position it is possible to palpate the difference between true abduction involving TFL and gluteus, or rotation, because of malcoordination between them, with gluteus being felt to 'come in' too late. If abduction is difficult with resistance, do same test without it (grade 3).

In the side-lying position there should be a vertical line from one ASIS to the other, to the table surface. True abduction takes place without any pelvic motion. If the pelvis is elevated during the test, quadratus is being used, and motion is taking place at the lumbosacral region.

If there is lateral rotation and flexion at the hip, TFL and iliopsoas are dominating the glutei. If abduction is very weak do the same test lying supine (Grade 2 or 1). It is also useful to perform TFL assessment as described in Chapter 4 (p.97).

Is Psoas Shortness Involved?

Janda says: 'The most important imbalance in the pelvic region is between the hip flexors and the trunk erectors,' (he calls this 'lower crossed syndrome'). He continues:

This imbalance causes an altered position of the pelvis producing stress in standing and walking, especially at L5–S1, producing pain and irritation. A similar imbalance occurs between the lateral corset muscles, gluteus medius and minimus and quadratus. Again L5–S1 will be irritated, this time in the sagittal plane.

Lewit says,

The thoraco-lumbar junction is the most unstable of the four major key transition regions as here two mobile structures meet, and the quality of the motion possible changes. To stabilise this region muscular forces are required (involving mainly iliopsoas, thoracic erector spinae, quadratus and rectus abdominus). Psoas spasm causes abdominal pain, flexion of the hip and typical antalgesic posture. If a number of these muscles are involved normalising one often corrects the others, as does treatment of the thoracolumbar restriction.

Cailliet provides the following guides as to the role of psoas in contraction:

- If the lumbar spine is fixed, contraction of the psoas results in flexion of the femur on the pelvis.
- If the femur is fixed the psoas insertion becomes the origin and the origin in turn becomes the insertion on the lumbar spine. Shortening in this situation causes traction on the anterior lumbar spine and an increase in lumbar lordosis.

This view is disputed by osteopathic researchers (Kappler, Fryett) who state that chronic contracture of psoas muscles (usually) results in loss of normal lumbar A-P curve with flattening and even reversal of that curve. Fryett goes on:

> In unilateral psoitis the muscle shortens and works from both ends with the result that the patient is drawn forward and sidebent to the involved side. The ilium on that side rotates backwards on the sacrum and the thigh is everted.
>
> Psoas is extremely sensitive to strain and toxaemias such as dead teeth, prostatitis, gonorrhoea, common cold etc... the primary predisposing cause is usually an articular lesion at 1st or 2nd lumbar.
>
> When both muscles are involved, and the tensions are equal, the patient is drawn forward with the lumbar curve locked against backward bending and side bending. Forward bending can usually increase though.

Flexion stress is the main mechanical cause of problems in psoas. If osteopathic research is right, diagnosis can therefore often be based on observation of A-P curve status, fixation of the upper lumbars in flexion, restricted in extension, being the hallmark.

If the lumbar A-P curve is normal this suggests that psoas is unlikely to be involved, *unless a paradoxical situation exists* (see below). Despite what Keppler and Fryett state above (i.e. that the spine goes into flexion if psoas is bilaterally short) a paradoxical, opposite, effect is also seen.

It there is marked erector spinae shortening together with marked bilateral tightness of iliopsoas the action of psoas switches to a dorsal direction; it no longer acts as a flexor of the spine but as an extensor, or rather it supports hyperlordosis of the lumbar segments. This was observed many times in cases of poliomyelitis (says Janda) and in this situation the patient can sit up with iliopsoas activity alone, without abdominal assistance.

So, the tighter the trunk erectors the more likely the psoas paradox is to exist. Such a patient will never strengthen the abdominals until the erectors are dealt with (due to constant reciprocal inhibition) at which time psoas reverts to being a lumbar flexor. *Psoas contraction bilaterally will show different clinical pictures depending on whether the erectors are overtight or normal.*

Psoas Symptoms

Symptoms of acute psoas dysfunction include the positional factors already mentioned, as well as pain which seems to start at the midline and lumbosacral area (where the majority of stress forces concentrate, producing increased extension, whcn lumbodorsal junction is fixed). Pain usually radiates laterally and abdominal pain is common. As psoas contracts, if the upper lumbars become fixed in flexion, the lumbosacral area builds up accommodating stresses, the posture alters accordingly. As postural side shift occurs, pain develops on the side of the greater instability in the gluteal and SI regions. Therapy is often misguidedly directed at the lumbosacral and sacroiliac regions, making matters worse (Keppler, Fryett).

Examination of Psoas, Including Modified Thomas Test

Exercise 38. Patient stands at end of table with back to it, one knee and hip are flexed which patient clasps close to stomach. Patient lies backwards with coccyx close to end and avoiding lordosis.

a. Free thigh should be horizontal to table; if not psoas is short.
b. Calf should be almost at right angle to thigh; if not rectus femoris is short. If this is so and patient's knee is passively bent to 90° there will be involuntary flexion of hip.
c. If there is groove in lateral thigh and patella deviates laterally, suspect TFL shortening. If this is so and leg is adducted, hip will flex involuntarily.

Place patient's arms above head (supine) observe if length is equal.

Exercise 39. Patient should be in the same position, both legs hanging down. Stand between your patient's legs, their feet pressed against your lateral calf, your hands resting on their thighs, have them try to 'lift' you from the floor *with their feet*. Assess relative strength. Compare with tightness test. If a psoas is both tight and strong, stretching is called for. If tight and weak deal with other factors (such as tight erector spinae muscles) first. If psoas is short, the modified Thomas test proves it (this is usually confirmed by overarm test for length equality – the side of the short arm is on the side of the short psoas).

Stretching is achieved by hip extension with lumbar spine stabilized (isometric muscle energy methods).

Observation of psoas incompetence shows:

- Ribcage tips forwards and down as abdominal recti pull on it.
- Rhomboids become incompetent.
- Body becomes flexed at groin, i.e. psoas is 'glued down' as it crosses pelvic brim preventing truly erect posture. (Psoas always produces aberrations around the groin when in trouble).

On spinal flexion psoas should 'fall back' if recti and psoas are interacting well. This shows as a flattening of the stomach rather than a bulging, as you bend forwards.

Exercise 40 a. Have patient lie on the floor and draw the legs up, together, dragging the heels and keeping them together. If the small of the back arches, psoas is inadequate to its job. Waistline should 'fall back'.

b. Have the patient lie on the back and extend legs skywards. Does the belly mound up? If so then the recti and psoas are not in balance. A competent psoas should allow raising of legs to the vertical position without hardening of recti.

Cailliet reminds us (*Low Back Pain*) that SLR to 30° is accomplished by iliopsoas which confirms Rolf's view. Beyond 30° the abdominals can take over SLR as iliopsoas becomes less effective. Cailliet suggests SLR exercises aimed at abdominal strengthening should only ever begin from the 30° position to minimize stress on the lumbar spine and psoas. Lewit says that attention to tight erector spinae would take care of lack of tone in the abdominals without much need for exercise of this sort.

Is Piriformis Shortness Involved?
Piriformis involvement in any pelvic or lower extremity problem may be assumed if there exists:

- Pain near greater trochanter
- Pain in inguinal area
- Local tenderness over piriformis tendon and muscle
- SI joint pain on *opposite side*
- Unilateral splay foot attitude on affected side
- Sciatic type pain to knee
- Pain unrelieved by position, patient is happiest when upright and moving
- Limitation of internal rotation of leg, producing pain in hip region
- *Affected side short*
- Pain and limitation of motion at T10 & T11
- Tension in area of T3 and T4
- Pain and limited motion at C2 on opposite site to dysfunction and concomitant atlanto-occipital lesion on same side due to shortness of affected leg (treatment of the secondary lesions will be ineffective until piriformis is corrected).

The symptoms of piriformis syndrome are commonly as follows: persistent, severe, radiating low back pain extending from sacrum to hip joint, over gluteal region and posterior portion of upper leg to the popliteal space. Change of position usually does not relieve symptoms, sitting, squatting, lying and standing all being uncomfortable. The buttock is extremely tender. There is usually persistent external rotation of the leg, which appears short. These symptoms in the absence of the short leg sign indicate some other factor than piriformis, as a rule.

The spinal and pelvic pattern seen is usually as follows: right piriformis contraction produces left oblique axis rotation of sacrum; sacral base on the right goes anterior in relation to PSIS; sulcus overlying the spine is palpated as being deeper; apex of sacrum moves left of midline and posteriorly at level of PSIS; sulcus on left side appears and palpates as more shallow because of posterior movement of sacrum.

Mitchell suggests an assessment of relative strength and shortness of external rotators of the hip in which:

a. patient is prone, knees flexed and ankles are grasped and abducted to place hips in maximum available internal rotation. Operator compares range of motion available (degree of movement from midline) without undue force (passive range). Equality of rotation indicates no imbalance. Inequality could mean tightness one side or weakness on the other.

b. Operator stands at foot of table, between legs, knees flexed to 90°, stabilizing the lower leg at limit of range of motion of internal rotation of hips. Patient tries to bring ankles to the midline against resistance, externally rotating the hip. Operator grades relative strength.

If evidence of (a) and (b) are supportive of shortness on one side, without undue weakness in the opposite piriformis, the shortness should be treated (i.e. inequality of length is evident in test (a) and the side of no limitation in test (a) shows itself to be not unduly weak in test (b)). Piriformis shortness can lead to pudendal nerve and blood supply disruption and serious problems involving the genitalia in both sexes, as well as extreme pain on intercourse in women due to leg position.

Exercise 41. The full assessment sequence for piriformis should be as follows:

a. Observe for shortness and external rotation.

b. Palpate piriformis insertion area for sensitivity (found where a line from the ASIS to the ischium intersects one from the PSIS to the trochanter).

c. Assess the relative freedom of internal and external rotation of the leg (supine).

d. Assess the passive range of motion of internal rotation of the hip (patient prone) and then relative weakness from same position (Mitchell, as above).

e. Patient should be supine. Cross the suspected leg over extended other leg, and apply medial pressure in order to stretch piriformis. Pain behind the trochanter suggests involvement.

f. Use the guidelines in the note on p.55 to see whether the pain is muscular or joint in origin. Do passive and active motions in opposite directions produce the pain? Does stretching of the muscle produce the pain?

g. Look at sacral landmarks to see if this coincides with what is anticipated in piriformis dysfunction (see notes above).

h. If there is sciatic pain on straight leg raising does it vanish with external rotation (if so piriformis is involved)?

By working your way through the various tests associated with short leg/long leg problems, as described by various experts, and by also evaluating (palpating and observing where appropriate) associated pelvic and muscular involvement you should have had the opportunity to assess your palpatory and observational skills to a great degree.

Assessing Dural Restriction

Dr John Upledger (*Craniosacral Therapy*) explains how difficult it is to prescribe techniques used to localize restrictions imposed upon the spinal dural tube. It is not that the techniques themselves are difficult, it is describing them that is hard. The dura is firmly attached along the entire circumference of the forearm magnum as well as to the posterior bodies of the second and third cervical vertebrae. From there it is free until it reaches the second sacral segment (anterior portion). After this it attaches, via the filum terminale to the periosteum of the coccyx. Adhesions and restriction can occur, not only at the points of attachment, but anywhere along its length, notably at intervertebral foramena. Simultaneous testing of motion at the occiput and sacrum allows mobility of the dura to be assessed, movements of which will be synchronous, if normal mobility exists. Any 'lag' of one bone or the other indicates restriction.

Upledger suggests palpating the motion in these bones simultaneously as the patient lies supine. If a normal synchronous motion is palpated he advocates experimentally slightly inhibiting the motion of either the occiput or the sacrum with one hand, and noting the effect on the motion being perceived by the other hand.

If, in the assessment, dural drag is presumed, due to a 'lag' between the occipital and sacral motions, he asks you to see whether you can tell whether this drag is coming from one end or the other, or from somewhere in between (within the dural tube or on one of its spinal nerve sleeves)? A further assessment is possible by simply introducing gentle occipital traction (patient supine) in order to cause the mobile dural tube to move gently towards you. If there is any restriction in this 'glide', ask yourself how far down the tube the restriction is taking place.

Light traction pulls on the tube closer to your hands (upper cervical) and as force builds up, this influences the dura further down its course. With practice one segment at a time can be 'palpated' by gently stretching the dura. Of course traction from the sacral end is also possible in the same manner.

Upledger describes an effective training exercise which sharpens perception of such restrictions as may be present: take a good length of cling-film and flatten this along the length of a smooth, clean table. The polyethylene will cling to the surface to a degree, offering resistance to any movement along the length of the table as you pull on one end.

Initially he suggests you apply traction and see how much effort is required to cause some movement of the film. After establishing this he suggests placing an object (a glass of water) on the film before repeating the exercise to see how the degree of traction needs to be increased, to take account of the weight of the object. Repetitive exercising in this way, with the weight in different positions, will increase perception of how motion is restricted in different localities.

After becoming familiar with variations in position of restriction, he suggests you perform a series of exercises of this sort blindfolded (someone else places the object on the film) to see whether you can assess how far down the table the object has been placed, purely by assessing the resistance in the film as you pull on it. 'You will be surprised how quickly you can develop accuracy at touching the object which offers the restriction to your traction while you are blindfolded.'

After this, retest the 'feel' of dural resistance with the patient supine, as you apply light traction to the occiput or sacrum.

Chapter 8

Visceral Palpation and Breathing Function Assessment

There is really only one way to learn visceral palpation and that is to achieve a high degree of palpatory literacy and to practise, practise, practise. And there is much to practise on. In their classic text, *Bodymechanics* (1935), Goldthwaite and his colleagues described the changes which were commonly found in association with a loss of diaphragmatic efficiency and abdominal ptosis:

- Breathing dysfunction and restrictions develop.
- There is drag on the fascia supporting the heart, displacing this organ and resulting in traction on the aorta. Nerve structures supplying the heart are similarly stressed mechanically.
- The cervical fascia is stretched (recall that this can lead to distortion anywhere from the cranium to the feet, as the fascia is continuous throughout the body).
- Venous stasis develops below the diaphragm (pelvic organs and so on) as its pumping action is inhibited and diminished, leading to varicose veins and haemorrhoids.
- The stomach becomes depressed and tilted, affecting its efficiency mechanically.
- The oesophagus becomes stretched, as does the coeliac artery. Symptoms ranging from hiatus hernia to dyspepsia and constipation become more likely.
- The pancreas is mechanically affected, interfering with its circulation. The liver is tilted backwards, there is inversion of the bladder, the support of the kidneys is altered and the colon and intestines generally become mechanically crowded and depressed (as does the bladder). None of these can therefore function well.
- The prostate becomes affected due to circulatory dysfunction and increased pressure, making hypertrophy more likely. Similarly menstrual irregularities become more likely.
- Increased muscular tension becomes a drain on energy, leading to fatigue which is aggravated by inefficient oxygen intake and poor elimination of wastes.
- Spinal and rib restrictions become chronic making this problem worse.
- Postural joints become stressed, leading to spinal, hip, knee and foot dysfunction, increasing wear and tear.

All these changes are palpable. And all are correctable, if caught early enough. A more precise examination of mechanical visceral dysfunction is now available through texts such as the highly recommended *Visceral Manipulation* (Jean-Pierre Barral and Pierre Mercier) which gives a host of directions, instructions and useful hints for anyone interested in this area of palpation and treatment. These British-trained osteopaths have developed the art of visceral palpation and manipulation to a very high level of expertise, constantly maintaining the precepts of osteopathic philosophy and practice. There is no way that it will be possible in the space available in this chapter to do more than indicate the sort of palpation exercise required to start emulating their work.

In their opening chapter they outline what we need to know about visceral motility and mobility:

> There is an inherent axis of rotation in each of these motions (mobility and motility). In healthy organs, the axes of mobility and motility are generally the same. With disease, they are often at variance with one another, as certain restrictions affect one motion more than another. What a surprise it was for us to discover that the axes of motion reproduce exactly those of embryological development! Neither preconceived ideas nor hypotheses directed this research. The discovery of this phenomenon was purely empirical, and tends to confirm the idea that 'cells do not forget'.

The various motions concurrently acting in the body are numerous and potentially confusing as palpation takes place. Visceral motion is influenced by:

1. The somatic nervous system (body movement, muscular tone and activity, posture). An example by Barral and Mercier is of the motion of the liver during flexion, as it slides forwards over the duodenum and the hepatic flexure of the colon below. Similar motions occur in all viscera determined by the particular support they have and their anatomical relationships.
2. Autonomic nervous system, including diaphragmatic motion, cardiac pulsation and motion as well as peristaltic activity. Clearly these automatic motions influence those organs closely associated in terms of locality as well as some at a distance (diaphragmatic motion, 24,000 times daily, influences and to some extent moves – or vibrates – all organs).
3. Craniosacral rhythm as we have seen in earlier chapters involves palpable movement throughout the body, most certainly including the viscera.

These 3 influences produce visceral mobility. And there is also inherent organ motility which, Barral and Mercier have indicated, relates very much to the embryological development phases. As an example the authors describe how during the development of the foetus the stomach rotates to the right in the transverse plane and clockwise in the frontal plane. The transverse rotation therefore orients the anterior lesser curve of the stomach to the right, and the greater posterior curvature to the left. The pylorus is therefore rotated superiorly and the cardia inferiorly.

The authors found that these directions 'remain inscribed in the visceral tissues' with motion occurring around an axis, a point of balance, as it moves further into the direction of embryological motion and then returns to neutral (very similar to what takes place in the craniosacral mechanisms during flexion and extension of the structures of the skull).

The motility cycle is divided into two phases which are termed *inspir* and *expir*. These are unrelated to the breathing cycle, being similar to the descriptions used in cranial osteopathy for cranial motion, flexion and extension. Inspir describes the inherent motion and expir the return to neutral afterwards (7 to 8 cycles per minute). An example of this is that the liver's inherent inspir phase involves rotation postosuperiorly (its mobility, as influenced by inhalation's diaphragmatic movement is almost exactly opposite, anteroinferior).

In palpation it is often easier to feel the expir phase (although inspir is more 'active' as there is less resistance to it) being a return to neutral. An additional vital, yet confusing, element is chronobiological influence. It is necessary to take account of the 'energy clock' initially described in Traditional Chinese Medicine (TCM) but now universally recognized as describing very pertinent changes in physiological function through the 24-hour period. The peak for energy circulation through the associated meridians in TCM is as follows:

- For the lungs it is between 3.00 and 5.00 a.m.
- Large intestines 5.00 and 7.00 a.m.
- Stomach 7.00 to 9.00 a.m.
- Spleen 9.00 to 11.00 a.m.
- Heart 11.00 am to 1.00 p.m.
- Small Intestine 1.00 p.m. to 3.00 p.m.
- Bladder 3.00 to 5.00 p.m.
- Kidney 5.00 to 7.00 p.m.
- Pericardium 7.00 to 9.00 p.m.
- Triple Burner 9 to 11 p.m.
- Gall Bladder 11 p.m. to 1 a.m.
- Liver 1 to 3 a.m.

Other monthly, seasonal and annual cycles require consideration in visceral palpation/manipulation.

Just as joints have articulations, so do viscera have 'articulations'. These are made of sliding surfaces (meninges in the CNS, pleura in the lungs, peritoneum in the abdominal cavity and pericardium in the heart) as well as a system of attachments (including ligaments, intercavity pressure, various folds of peritoneal structures forming containment and supportive elements). Unlike most joints, few muscular forces directly move organs.

Factors such as adhesions and fixations within the supporting tissues and 'articulations' influence visceral motion negatively, as does overall displacement via ptosis (sagging or laxity), the influence of muscular restriction through spasm as well as anything which disturbs the associated rhythmic factors in the body, such as the diaphragm's action.

Barral and Mercier suggest that there are three elements involved in evaluation of visceral function, and these are the traditional ones of palpation (which informs as to tone of the walls of the visceral cavity), percussion (which informs about the position and size of the organ in question) and auscultation (which informs as to factors such as circulation of air, blood and secretions such as bile).

These authors stress the importance of the influence on visceral function of muscular activity and urge mobility tests to identify dysfunction in the musculoskeletal system. They however state 'We believe that visceral restrictions are the causative lesions much more frequently than are musculoskeletal restrictions.'

How do you palpate an organ for mobility? By precise movements, say Barral and Mercier. In order to do this though you need to know the normal movements of the organ in question. They give an example of the liver which, 'you literally lift up to appreciate the elasticity of its supporting structures and the extent of its movement'. Mobility assessment (which provides information as to elasticity, laxity/ptosis, spasm and structural injury of muscular or ligamentous supports) requires less skill than does finer evaluation of inherent motility and variations in it from the norm.

How do you palpate organs for motility? The most effective method for evaluating motility, say Barral and Mercier, is the method described by Rollin Becker D.O. (see Chapter 5 p.126) in which the hand 'listens' for information. This is how the French osteopaths describe application of Becker's work to this task:

> Place your hand over the organ to be tested, with a pressure of 20–100g, depending on the depth of the organ. In some cases the hand can adapt itself to the form of the organ. The hand is totally passive, but there is an extension of the sense of touch used during this examination. Let the hand passively follow what it feels – a slow movement of feeble amplitude which will show itself, stop and then begin again (7 to 8 per minute in health). This is visceral motility.

It is desirable, then, after a few cycles, to estimate elements such as frequency, amplitude and direction of the motility. The advice is very much as given by Becker, Upledger, Smith and others (see Chapter 5). Do not have preconceived ideas as to what will be felt. Trust what you feel. Empty the mind and let the hand listen. (Both organs of a pair should be assessed and compared.)

One visceral palpation exercise – for motility (based on the work of Barral and Mercier) is suggested below. Those exercises relating to Becker's work, as outline in Chapter 5, should have been performed satisfactorily before performing this exercise. Study of visceral manipulation and attendance at seminars and workshops covering this subject is suggested for those keen to explore this subtle and rewarding field.

Exercise 1. Palpation for liver motility. Patient is supine. The examiner (seated or standing on the right of the patient, facing him/her) places the right hand over the lower ribs, molding to their curve, covering the outer aspect of the liver.

Lay the left hand over the right, and allow the mind to become still. If it helps visualize the liver.

Remember that you are trying to assess the return to neutral (expir phase of the motility cycle), which means that the actual direction of active motion would be the opposite to that palpated in this phase. Barral and Mercier suggest this expir phase to be the easiest for the beginner to palpate.

During this expir phase three simultaneous motions may be felt:

- On the frontal plane a counter-clockwise motion from right to left around the sagittal axis (of your hand and therefore the liver). This takes the palm of the hand towards the umbilicus.
- In the sagittal plane the superior part of the hand should rotate anteroinferiorly around a transverse axis through the middle of your hand.
- In the transverse plane the hand rotates to the left around a vertical axis bringing the palm off the body as the fingers seem to press more closely.

Each of these planes of movement can be assessed separately before they are simultaneously assessed, providing a clear picture of liver motility in the expir phase of the cycle (inspir is the exact opposite).

Try performing this palpation exercise with the eyes closed and also have the patient periodically hold the breath for 20 second periods to see whether this gives you a less confused feeling of motion. Remember also Becker's method of assessment (Chapter 5) using his elbows or forearm as a fulcrum. Use this to enhance palpatory sensitivity and see whether it in fact increases your perception.

Respiration Assessment

Lewit (*Manipulation in Rehabilitation of the Motor System*) has synthesized much of the current knowledge about respiratory influence on body mechanics, and describes useful methods for assessing its efficiency and coordination:

> Thinking of breathing, one naturally has in mind the respiratory system. Yet it is the locomotor system that makes the lungs work, and the locomotor system that has to coordinate the specific respiratory movements with the rest of the body's locomotor activity. This task is so complex that it would be a miracle if disturbances did not occur.

The consequences of respiratory dysfunction can be very profound indeed, often leading to hyperventilation (see p.204) with its repercussions in the area of anxiety production, phobic states and panic attacks, as well as massive interference in energy cycles leading to chronic fatigue. The negative effects of poor respiratory function on cardiac and circulatory function add a further dimension to its importance. From the viewpoint of body mechanics, sound respiratory function has surprising influences.

Muscular activity is enhanced by inspiration and inhibited by expiration, in general. There are exceptions such as the abdominal muscles which are facilitated by forced exhalation. Flexion of the cervical and lumbar spines is enhanced by maximum exhalation whereas flexion of the thoracic spine is enhanced by maximum inspiration, and these phases of respiration can be usefully employed in mobilization (and assessment including palpation) of this region.

A further influence on spinal mechanics of respiration is described by Lewit:

> The most surprising effect of inspiration and expiration is the alternating facilitation and inhibition of individual segments of the spinal column during sidebending, discovered by Gaymans (1980). It can be regularly shown that during sidebending, resistance increases in the cervical as well as the thoracic regions, in the even segments (occiput-atlas, C2 etc and again T2, T4 etc) during inspiration; during expiration we gain the mobilizing effect in these segments. Conversely, resistance increases in the odd segments during expiration (C1, C3 etc T3, T5 etc). There is a neutral zone between C7 and T1.

Inspiration increases resistance to movement in the atlas-occiput region in all directions, while expiration eases its motion in all directions, a most useful piece of information, of value during manipulation or assessment/palpation of motion.

Where maximum muscular effort is required we tend to neither inhale nor exhale, but to hold the inhaled breath (Valsalva manoeuvre). This achieves postural stability (no facilitation of spinal motion in any segments) at the cost of momentary loss of respiratory function. The diaphragm has therefore been described (according to Lewit) as 'a respiratory muscle with postural function' while the abdominal muscles are 'postural muscles with respiratory function'. These comments highlight the role of the diaphragm in supporting the spine. As Lewit explains, the abdominal cavity is a fluid-filled space which is not compressible just as long as the abdominal muscles and the perineum are contracted (the shout of the judo wrestler, ski jumper and weight lifter all attest to this enhanced stability being used).

A further stabilizing feature is the fact that as we rise on our toes the diaphragm contracts (at start of a race, when jumping for example) this being interpreted as a postural reaction. Lewit sees inspiration as largely dependent on contraction of the diaphragm which lifts the lower ribs just as long as the central tendon is supported by counterpressure from sound abdominal muscles. This, he says, is the only explanation of the widening of the thorax from below (see also Latey's assessments of this function in Chapter 10).

The thorax must be widened from below to achieve postural stability during respiration, never raised from above. Therefore the shoulders, clavicles and upper ribs are not lifted but rotate slightly to accommodate the movement from below as the thorax widens. This does not happen when supine or on all fours, where no postural stabilizing effect is needed, and pure abdominal respiration becomes physiologically normal, with the abdomen bulging while its wall remains relaxed.

These preliminary explanations are necessary to understand what we should look for when respiratory dysfunction is active. What then should be observe and palpate?

1. Inactive abdominal muscles are clearly undesirable for respiratory and postural normality, for the spine then loses its diaphragmatic support. The abdominal tone can be assessed with the patient seated and relaxed. There should be no flabbiness on palpation. On stooping from the standing position the abdominals should be felt to contract.

Recall that Janda has shown (see Chapter 4) that tight erector spinae muscles will effectively reciprocally inhibit the abdominal musculature, and that no amount of toning exercise can restore normalcy until the erectors spinae group are stretched and normalized. The test for abdominal muscle efficiency involves having the patient sit up from the supine position while knees and hips are flexed. In order to have coordinated action from the glutei (maximus) in this action the heels may press *backwards* against a firm cushion or support. If this is difficult then lying backwards from a seated position will train the abdominals.

The spine is flexed first and one segment at a time is laid on the table/floor without raising the feet from the floor. If the feet start to leave the floor, stop the movement backwards at this point and slowly return to the upright seated position. Keep repeating the lay back, trying to increase the distance travelled before the feet start to rise.

2. The thorax must be seen to widen from below on inhalation. Also, when sitting flexed or lying prone, there must be a visible ability to breathe 'into' the posterior thoracic wall. This is evidenced by the respiratory 'wave' described in Chapter 7 (p.160, exercise 20).

Where this wave is absent – starting in the low lumbars and progressing throughout inhalation up to the cervico-dorsal junction – there will be palpable restrictions in the thoracic spine due to the absence of the mobilizing effect of the breathing function.

3. The most obvious evidence of poor respiratory function is the raising of the upper chest structures by means of contraction of the upper fixators of the shoulder and the auxiliary cervical muscles (upper trapezius, levator scapulae, scalenes, sternomastoid and so on). This is both inefficient as a means of breathing and the cause of stress and overuse to the cervical structures. It is clearly evident (see below) when severe but may require a deep inhalation to show itself, if only slight.

Exercise 2. Assessing respiratory function.
1. Patient seated, stand behind and place hands, facing forwards, over lower ribs. Patient inhales. Is there a lateral widening?
   Or do your hands seem to be raised upwards?
   The hands should move apart, but they will be felt to rise if

inappropriate breathing is being performed.

Does one side seem to move more than the other?

If so local restrictions or muscle tensions are involved.

2. Rest the hands over the upper shoulder area, fingers facing forwards. On inhalation do the hands rise?

Does the clavicle rise on inhalation?

Neither the clavicle nor your hands should rise, even on forced inhalation. While in this position assess whether one side moves more than the other. If so local restrictions or muscle tensions are involved.

3. Observe the upper trapezius as they curve towards the neck.

Are they convex (bowing outwards)?

If so these (called 'gothic' shoulders) are very taut and probably accompany inappropriate breathing, lifting the upper ribs (along with scalenes, sternomastoid and levator scapulae).

Palpate these muscles, and test them for shortness (see Chapter 4).

4. Palpate the abdomen, still with the patient seated, as she inhales deeply.

Does it (slightly) bulge on inhalation? This is normal. In some instances, breathing is so faulty that the abdomen is drawn in in inhalation and pushed outwards on exhalation.

5. Go back to the first position, hands on the sides of the lower ribs.

Feel the degree of contraction on exhalation.

Does this seem to be a complete exhalation?

Or does the patient not quite get the last breath exhaled before commencing the next inhalation?

If so this leads to retention of excessive levels of tidal air, preventing a full inhalation. Inhalation efficiency can be said to depend on the completeness of the exhalation.

6. Ask the patient to take as long as possible to breathe in completely. How long did it take?

If less than 5 seconds there is probably dysfunction.

Next, after a complete inhalation, ask them to take as long as possible to exhale, breathing out slowly all the time (not a fast exhalation followed by a period during which nothing happens). This should also take no less than 5 seconds, although people with dysfunction, or who hyperventilate and those in states of anxiety, often fail to take even as long as 3 seconds to inhale or exhale.

Time the complete cycle if breathing. This should take not less than 10 seconds in good function.

7. Patient lies supine, knees flexed. Rest a hand lightly just above the umbilicus and have them inhale deeply.

Does your hand move towards the ceiling?

Are the abdominal muscles relaxed?

Or did the hand actually drop towards the floor on inhalation?

The answer to the first two questions should be 'yes', and to the third a definite 'no'.

If the abdomen rises, was this the first part of the respiratory mechanism to move, or did it inappropriately follow an initial movement of the upper or lower chest? Paradoxical breathing such as this involves the mechanism being used in just such an uncoordinated manner.

8. Lie the patient prone and observe the wave as inhalation occurs, moving upwards in a fan-like manner from the lumbars to the base of the neck. This wave can be observed by watching the spinous processes or the paraspinal musculature, or palpated by a feather-light touch on the spine or paraspinal structures.

Whatever restrictions or uncoordinated movements you observe or palpate during this exercise can now usefully be related to findings of spinal restrictions, rib dysfunction (Chapter 7), respiratory and postural muscular shortening as well as trigger point activity – especially in the intercostal muscles (Chapter 4), postural imbalance, pelvic dysfunction and short leg anomalies (Chapter 7), emotional involvement (Chapter 10). Integrating the various components of palpation as described throughout the book will help to sharpen the palpatory literacy which is the objective of the work.

Special Note

About Hyperventilation

The effect of over-breathing is to reduce swiftly the levels of carbon dioxide in the blood, altering the acid-alkaline balance and thus producing changes in the way nerves interact with each other, resulting in a variety of unpleasant symptoms.

Many studies have concentrated on the widespread problem of over-breathing. Much of this has related to its connection with anxiety states in which it can lead to acute phobic states, accompanied by panic attacks of an incapacitating nature. The symptoms most often associated with hyperventilation include giddiness, dizziness, faintness, numbness in the upper limbs, face or trunk, loss of consciousness (fainting), visual disturbances in which blurring or even temporary loss of vision is experienced, headaches of a general nature often accompanied by nausea and frequently diagnosed as migraine, inability to walk properly (ataxia) as well as trembling and head noises. A number of symptoms often associated with heart function can become apparent during or after hyperventilation, including palpitation, chest discomfort, difficulty in taking a deep breath, insomnia, fatigue, weakness in the limbs and much more.

Of patients diagnosed with hyperventilation more than half are found to be undergoing stress, related to marriage, work or finance. Hyperventilation is not, however, always associated with psychiatric stress and this is made clear in correspondence in the *Journal of the Royal Society of Medicine* (November 1987) in which it is stated that, 'The underlying disorder (of hyperventilation) may be psychiatric, organic, a habit disorder or a combination of these.'

How to Deal with Hyperventilation

In most instances of hyperventilation a combination exists of a learned pattern of breathing coming into operation in response to real or assumed stressful situations. This is usually found to co-exist alongside severely contracted muscles relating to the rib cage, spinal regions and the diaphragm area. These are readily palpable or observable.

There is as we know a tendency to 'lock' our emotional states into our muscles (see Chapter 10). You only have to sit quietly and imagine a strong emotion such as fear or hatred or anger, for subtle yet perceptible changes to be felt in the muscles of the neck, shoulders, chest, pit of stomach and so on.

If this were not just an imagined emotion but a strongly held one which lasted for many months or years, as is all too often the case, chronic shortening and tension would develop in many muscles of the body. These could include: scalenes, trapezius (upper fibres), levator scapulae, sternomastoid, pectorals, intercostals, spinal erectors, abdominals. Such changes are a common feature amongst people who are chronically fatigued, since the combination of energy wastage, through long-held tension, and reduced oxygenation due to impaired respiratory function, can produce profound fatigue.

Muscles which are chronically hypertonic, shortened or contracted, cannot function normally and this is usually the case in people who hyperventilate; it seems they have learned to over-breathe excessively in response to what are not really stressful situations.

It is a perfectly normal to hyperventilate when excessive demands are required of the body. If however this response occurs inappropriately, in the face of a perceived but unreal crisis, such as exists when we are unnaturally anxious about something then the sequence of over-breathing would lead to imbalanced blood gas levels, changes in acidity/alkalinity and the whole sequence of hyperventilation symptoms listed. This can become an habitual method of responding to all minor stress situations leading to the complete misery of phobic states compounded by panic attacks and virtual incapacity and inability to function.

Such people respond well to breathing re-training and recognition of the fact that if they use their newly acquired slow breathing techniques in the face of a stressful (real or imagined) situation they can stop the symptoms because they simply will not hyperventilate. Correction of hyperventilation therefore should involve a threefold approach:

1. Learn not to respond to stress in the habitual way. This requires insights which may only be available from a good counsellor or psychotherapist. Relaxation techniques are a part of this.
2. Learn correct breathing techniques to use, especially when confronted by a frightening situation.
3. Normalize the machinery which governs breathing by bodywork and exercises, this conserves energy and allows normal function. The result of such an approach is a lessened waste of energy, increased functional ability in relation to breathing, and far fewer symptoms.

Chapter 9

Palpation without Touching the Physical Body (Therapeutic Touch)

Clearly anyone holding their hands above the surface of the body is not really palpating or manipulating the physical tissues themselves. However, the boundary between what we take to be the physical and something distinctly palpable above the surface, requires investigation. As we can see from Fritz Smith's work (and that of other 'energy' workers, see Chapter 5) it helps if we can 'visualize' an energy field/body when working in this as yet ill-defined area. Is there any evidence to support such subtle concepts?

Therapeutic Touch, as developed by Dolores Krieger, is a modern derivative of the laying on of hands which involves barely touching the patient's body, or the holding of hands away from the body surface, with an intent to help or heal. This method is now taught to members of the nursing profession worldwide, and recent research has validated its therapeutic value.

A fascinating, if somewhat inexplicable benefit, under controlled conditions, was reported in Volume X, number 2 of *Cooperative Connection* (Spring 1989) in an article entitled *'Effects of Therapeutic Touch on Tension Headache Pain'* by E. Keller and M. Bzdek. Sixty volunteers with tension headaches were divided randomly into two groups and were treated either with Therapeutic Touch – in which 5 minutes of non-touching energy balancing with healing intent was applied – or received 5 minutes of apparently identical methodology (hand position the same and so on) but with the therapist deliberately concentrating on mental arithmetic during the treatment.

Both groups were asked to sit quietly and breathe deeply during the real and placebo sessions, and *no physical contact was used on either group*.

Standard McGill-Melzack pain assessment questionnaires were used before, immediately after and 4 hours after each treatment or placebo treatment. 90 per cent of those exposed to Therapeutic Touch experienced sustained reduction in intensity in headache pain with an average of 70 per cent pain reduction, twice the average achieved immediately after Therapeutic Touch.

Dummy Therapeutic Touch (placebo) reduced pain in 80 per cent of patients but only by a level of 37 per cent for a shorter duration, since half the placebo group resorted to medication in the 4 hour period after, as compared with only 5 of the Therapeutic Touch group.

So what did the therapist actually do? Keller and Bzdek:

> The intervention began with the researcher centering herself into a meditative quiet and making conscious intent to help the subject. She then passed her hands 6 to 12 inches from the subject without physical contact to assess the energy field... and to redirect areas of accumulated tensions out of the field. She then let her hands rest around (not on) the head or solar plexus in areas of energy imbalance or deficit and directed life energy to the subject.

Those who do not, thus far, use such methods might care to think more about just what happens under these conditions, and to learn how to 'feel' the fluctuations in energy, something which is apparently palpable with practice.

As part of an attempt to achieve this, and to understand the mechanics of such interventions we will now assess the methods recommended by a number of experts in this field for palpating and treating, using 'energy'.

Dr Dolores Krieger

During the 1960s a series of experiments was conducted involving enzymes, plants and animals, in which the 'laying on of hands' was demonstrated to have profoundly protective effects in the face of a variety of negative influences, ranging from a deficiency diet to irradiation. Anyone who wishes to read a succinct account of these should study *Vibrational Medicine* by Richard Gerber M.D.

It was following the publication of such research – specifically research indicating an increase in chlorophyll in plants nourished by water which had been 'treated' by healers by Dr Bernard Grad, of McGill University – that Dolores Krieger, a professor of nursing at New York University, began to investigate the human potential of these methods. It was reasoned that since chlorophyll was chemically identical to haemoglobin, except that in the former a magnesium atom exists instead of iron, it should be possible to improve haemoglobin levels in humans by similar means.

A healer who had been involved in the plant experiments 'magnetically charged' rolls of cotton batting for a group of sick people to keep with them, as well as conducting a laying on of hands. A year later these patients were compared with a control group who had received no such 'treatment' and were found by Dr Krieger to have significantly raised haemoglobin levels. This was confirmed in later experiments and led Dr Krieger to begin teaching her method, dubbed Therapeutic Touch, to senior nurses. By this time Krieger had become convinced that what was being manipulated was *prahna* (subtle energy) as described in Hindu and yogic tradition.

In its simplest terms the method was conceived as the balancing of the energy field of someone in whom it had become disrupted or weakened, either as a result of ill-health or as a predisposing factor to that ill-

health. Individuals who are basically healthy have an abundance of
energy and can use this to help those in whom it is disturbed, with
profoundly beneficial effects, both physically and emotionally.

The potential to apply this form of healing resides in us all, says
Krieger (her book *The Therapeutic Touch* is highly recommended) and
its use can be developed by simple exercises. Krieger states that its two
most noticeable effects are the eliciting of a profound, generalized
relaxation as well as being good at relieving pain. What is called for,
before practising or performing Therapeutic Touch, is a 'centering'
process in which you learn to find within yourself an inner reference of
stability.

Krieger says: 'Centering... can be thought of as a place of inner being,
a place of quietude within oneself where one can be truly integrated,
unified and focussed.' This place is well known to those who practise
meditation and deep relaxation. It cannot be found by effort or strain:
'It is a conscious direction of attention inwards, an ''effortless effort''
that is conceptual but that can be experiential.'

It is not within the scope of this text to teach the reader to find that
quiet state; numerous texts and tapes exist, as well as opportunities for
individual or group instruction which can all lead to this state of

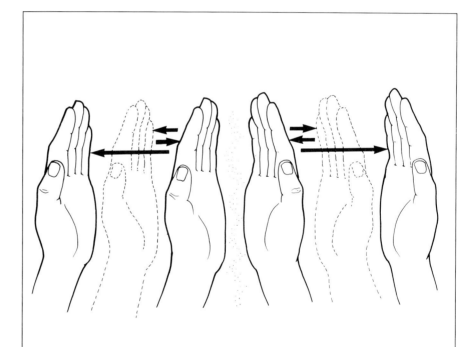

Fig. 33: Bring hands as close together as you can without the palms
touching each other. Then bring hands apart about two inches. Return
hands slowly to original position. Repeat, however, each time separate
the palms by an additional two inches, until they are finally eight inches
apart.

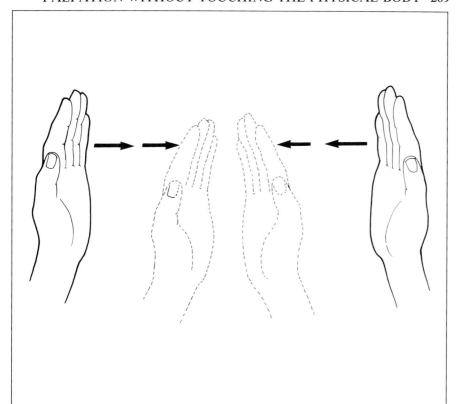

Fig. 34: When the hands are about eight inches apart, slowly bring them together. At every two inches test the field between your hands for a sense of bounciness or elasticity.

'balance, of equipoise, and of quietude that marks the experience of centering'. Once the therapist has achieved this, Krieger provides clear guidelines as to how we should begin palpating energy variables.

Exercise 1. Centre yourself and sit comfortably with both feet on the floor and place your hands so that the palms face each other. Your elbows should be held away from your trunk, the lower arms unsupported by anything. Bring the palms as close together as you can without actually allowing them to touch (perhaps as close as under a quarter of an inch). Slowly separate your hands to a gap of around 2 inches and then return them to the first position (a quarter inch gap). Next take them 4 inches apart and then slowly return them to the first position. Now go to a six inch gap (always very slowly) and come again to the first position.

Do you feel anything as the hands come close together?

A build up of 'pressure' in that small space perhaps?

Or do you feel any other sensation, such as a tingling or vibration?

Now take your palms 8 inches apart and this time do not bring them together again immediately, but rather do so in two inch increments; first to 6 inches apart, then 4 inches, 2 inches and finally the starting position. At each position stop and sense and 'test' what you can feel between your hands.

Do you sense a 'compression' of something between your hands? A 'bouncy' feeling?

If so, at what distance did this become apparent?

Take a minute or more to practise this exercise over and over again. Try to experience what you are feeling and note the characteristics of the elastic, bouncy, energy field you are holding between your hands. Do you feel heat, cold, tingling, pulsation, or something else altogether? This exercise can be practised whenever you have a spare moment until you are confident that what you feel is real and its characteristics become familiar.

Do it with your eyes closed or open, and see which is best for you. As Krieger says, 'You do not stop at your skin,' and this exercise proves this to you and allows you to develop the sensitivity for application of Therapeutic Touch.

Krieger provides a series of exercises which incrementally help you to become more aware of your own potentials in this field and her book is suggested as a working tool for those attracted to these methods.

Exercise 2. Having developed your skills in energy palpation, and having centred yourself, practise the following assessment of someone else's energy field. Have a 'model', or a real patient, who is sitting or lying. Place your hands 2 to 3 inches from their skin surface, perhaps starting at the head. Test the area to the left of the head and compare this with the right side. Scan from the top of the head, over the face to the chin, taking about 10 seconds to cover that area. Be aware of whatever you feel, changes in sensation, temperature and so on, but do not dwell on questions such as 'Did I or did I not feel something?' Simply sense what comes through your hands. Gradually move over the entire front of the body and then move to the back. Speed of movement is slow but steady.

When the complete scan is finished recheck any areas which seemed unusual, and recheck your first impressions. It may be that where there are significant variations in the energy field you will note temperature fluctuations through your hands. Or you may feel pressure changes, tingling, vibration, electric shock type sensations or pulsations instead. All may be significant.

Exercise 3. Relax and centre yourself and then scan the body of a partner or patient to see whether you feel any variations or changes in the texture and nature, of the energy field in the regions of the 'chakras', as described in Chapter 5 by Upledger.

Compare what you feel in the various chakra positions, with findings from 'normal' healthy energetic individuals and those who are unwell. See whether particular forms of ill-health relate to particular patterns of energy fluctuation.

Along with Dr Krieger's book a thoughtful and delightful introduction to energy medicine will be found in *Joy's Way* by Dr Joy. There is much which is similar to Krieger, but a good deal which is unique, with abundant material to help the reader in developing the ability to feel radiating energy fields as well as guidance in methods for 'transfer of energy to others'.

The Concepts of Brugh Joy M.D.

Joy describes what he teaches as Transformational Therapy and stresses that one set of exercises should be mastered before the next is attempted, describing them under the headings of:

1. Resonation circle
2. Exploration of greatly amplified musical sounds
3. Modified spiral meditation
4. Dyadic exercises
5. Triadic exercises
6. Hand scanning
7. Energy transfer.

It can be seen from this list alone that before getting to the place where Krieger starts, Joy suggests a good deal of work.

Joy's book is the best way of obtaining detailed directions in the first five of the above requirements. His description of hand scanning of chakras is worth studying as it gives a clear outline of his approach:

> During the hand-scanning phase of body-energy work the consciousness of the scanner must become totally receptive and his/her awareness must be centred entirely in the hand or hands. The witness state of consciousness is activated. One must be careful not to project what one thinks should be there into the space surrounding the person to be scanned. Instead the task is to explore that space in order to find out what is actually there. The hand that is acting as the detector is relaxed. The fingers should be slightly apart and may be bent, as in the classical ballet pose. A rigid flat hand, with the fingers held tightly together, is not nearly so effective a detector.

He suggests rolling up long sleeves exposing the skin of the forearm as this is often a more sensitive detector than the hand. He suggests beginners start with the right hand (if they are right handed) as it is hard to be efficient with both hands at first; both will eventually become suitably sensitive.

Speed of movement is important, as going too quickly prevents the mind from registering sensory input, and going too slowly allows the scanner's own energy to be reflected back from the body surface, so that all surfaces feel the same. A foot every two seconds is about the right speed (faster than Krieger's suggested speed of 10 seconds for the face alone).

A common sensation for the beginner is to feel 'overcharged', characterized by a tingle or pulsation or even an ache or pain. This prevents awareness of incoming stimuli. Joy suggests flicking the hands to relieve it or patting them on your own thigh. This may result from too much *trying*, which is not what is called for as you palpate the energy fields. The feeling has to be allowed to come through. Joy likens the process of learning this subtle palpation to what happens to medical students as they learn to detect heart murmurs:

> First they must learn where to centre their hearing awareness, because their ordinary hearing mechanism simply does not listen to the ranges where these murmurs can be heard. The same is true with the subtle sense of touch, at least at the beginning stages.

The distance from the body of the scanning hand should be 8 to 12 inches, says Joy, with the person to be scanned lying face upwards on a wooden bed or table (metal interferes with the energy field). All jewellery should be removed as should metal buckles and watches. The person being scanned should feel relaxed and free to move (to scratch) if they wish. Talking however should be discouraged.

Joy suggests a start be made by taking the pulse of the 'patient' in order to atune the scanner's consciousness to the patient's. With the other hand scanning can then begin over the chest and upper body and lower abdomens, as here the energy fields are strong and relatively easy to assess. He suggests the scanning hand starts off from the side of the body, beyond its edge, and moves into the area above the body and then out again for a contrast to be noted. As one becomes familiar with the feel of an energy field this is less necessary. He recommends the eyes be closed when working in this way, (as in skin or muscle palpation, for better focusing of the mind).

He gives a most important pointer when he says:

> The fields are not felt when the hand is held over them *but as the hand moves through them*. This principal is fundamental. *During a scan the hand must be in perpetual motion. It must pass in and out of the fields.*

Thus by 'slicing' through the energy fields at different levels its shape can be determined, its distance from the surface, its density and degree of 'health'.

Joy notes that after years of experience he can detect a field two or three times further from the body surface than can a beginner. At first simply registering the fact that an energy vortex exists over a chakra is a major step forward. The ones over the groin and the top of the head are relatively easy to detect. The variations in intensity should be registered as the scanning hand passes from chakra to chakra.

The region over the throat chakra requires that the patient hold their breath for a short while so that it does not confuse the scanning process. Practise in a group if possible so that the differences one from another are available to reinforce the learning process. After scanning the front of the body the patient turns over and the back is assessed in much the same manner.

Exercise 4. As an early exercise try scanning the back of the body without having first studied a 'map' of where the fields are most dense, and compare your findings with such a map later.

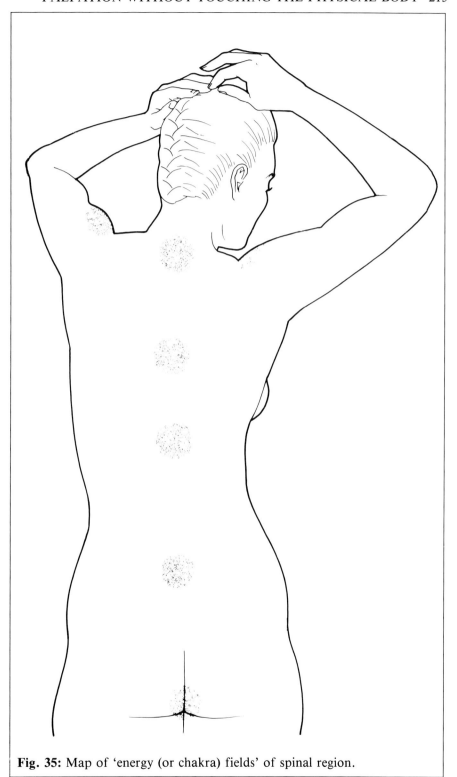

Fig. 35: Map of 'energy (or chakra) fields' of spinal region.

Exercise 5. With your patient lying face down palpate the energy fields on the front of the body by scanning under the table. Compare your findings with what you assessed when they were face upwards. The energy fields pass through the material of the table readily and are easily palpable at the same distance from the body as previously.

Before attempting to transfer energy (as in Therapeutic Touch), Joy suggests, it is essential to be able to scan in this way. He urges you to practise until all the chakras can be readily detected. It is not within the scope of this text to instruct in that phase of energy work, since detection of imbalances, and palpation in general, are our first objectives.

Following the guidelines of Krieger and Joy (as well as those given below) will open this area of palpation and those interested in carrying their knowledge further will find excellent help in the books quoted in this chapter.

Barbara Ann Brennan, in her fine explanation of her approach to healing through the human energy fields *Hands of Light*, explains what is known via scientific enquiry, and much that is still speculated upon, as she leads the reader through a series of training processes towards an ability to work in this area with confidence.

She describes a series of exercises which can assist in helping you to visualize the human aura (energy field) which she says is the manifestation of universal energy intimately involved in your (human) life. This is divided into various 'layers' or 'bodies' which interpenetrate each other, each succeeding one being of finer vibrational quality than the body which it surrounds and interpenetrates.

Exercise 6. If you are in a group make a circle in which you all hold hands. Sense a pulsating flow of energy if you can. In which direction is it travelling? (almost always from left to right around the circle). Ask your neighbour whether they feel the same thing.

Without moving anything, or altering the hand contact, Brennan asks you to 'stop the flow of energy'. Everyone in the circle should simultaneously hold this energy still for a short while before allowing it to flow again. This should be repeated several times as you feel the difference between energy flow and stillness.

Exercise 7. Sit opposite a partner with your palms facing theirs. Let any energy flow occur naturally. Then direct energy out of your left palm to their hand. Then stop this and bring energy into your right palm from their hand. Reverse and vary these flows and then stop it all together. Then attempt to 'push' energy out of both hands at the same time, and finally 'suck' energy into both simultaneously. A feeling of tickling, 'tingling or pressure', something like static electricity, indicates that the energy fields are touching the skin or that the fields are touching each other. 'Push, pull and stop are the three basic ways of manipulating energy in healing,' says Brennan.

Exercise 8. She then suggests you practise the exercise (1 above) given by Krieger as a first step in assessing the field between your hands, as you take them to varying distances apart and then slowly bring them together again until you feel the compressed energy in the space between your hands:

> If your hands are one and a quarter inches apart (when you feel the compression forces) you have touched your etheric body edges together (first layer of the aura). If your hands are three to four inches apart, you have touched the outside edges of your emotional body together (second layer of the aura).

She suggests you hold the hands about 7 inches apart and point your right index finger at the palm of the left hand and slowly draw circles with it. See whether you can feel this (eyes closed, centred) as a tickling sensation.

Exercise 9. Dim the room lights and hold your hands, fingertips pointing towards each other. The hands should be held in front of your face, about 2 feet away from your eyes. Have a plain white wall behind your hands. Relax your gaze and softly look at the space between your fingertips which should be an inch or two apart.

Moving the fingers towards and away from each other slightly, or taking one hand slightly upwards and the other down slightly, she asks that you note what you might be seeing between your fingers or around the hand. She suggests it will be the following in 95 per cent of people:

> Most people see a haze around the fingers and hands...it looks somewhat like the heat haze over a radiator. It is sometimes seen in various colours, such as a blue tint... The energy bodies pull like toffee between the fingers as the haze from each fingertip connects to the haze at the fingertip of the opposite hand.

As you move the fingertips so that different ones face each other, the haze may follow the old pattern before jumping back to the presently closest fingertip.

Brennan takes her reader through a host of gradually more complex exercises towards a full ability to palpate and manipulate the subtle energies around us all. Of practical value to those working in bodywork are her instructions regarding identification and interpretation of 'energy blocks' which she divides into six types. The way these are formed will depend largely, she believes, on variations of tactics we all adopt in our 'energetic defence systems', which we use to defend ourselves aggressively or passively, to repel incoming threatening forces. The end results of such defensive/protective strategies are palpable in the space just away from the body's 'energy blocks' which she categorizes as follows:

1. The 'blah' block. The result of 'depressing one's feelings' causing a stagnation of energy, with accumulation of fluid in the region involved. The physical body will be bloated at this region, the energy

having a low intensity rather than 'high energy'. The related emotions often have a despairing quality, or are associated with anger (in a blaming manner). Colitis or angina pectoris are examples of an end result. The 'feeling' of such a block is sticky, like mucus.

2. Compaction blocks are related to suppressed feelings, containing accumulated rage (volcanic, ready to explode). An 'ominous' feeling is associated with palpation or observation of such a block. Body fat or muscle accumulates in the regions affected. Diseases such as pelvic inflammatory disease may occur. The individual is usually aware of the suppressed rage, with a feeling of being trapped. Sexuality and a sense of humiliation may also be involved.

3. 'Mesh armour' is another pattern of block, used to help the individual avoid feelings, especially fear. The blocks are therefore shifted around when there is a challenge. Thus, if therapy releases associated tensions, they reappear elsewhere very rapidly. This type of block may not result in disease, the individual often appearing a 'perfect wife and mother', but with a vague sense of something lacking in life. Deep feelings are usually only tolerated for brief periods with intermittent crises occurring (sudden illness, affair, accident) as a pattern of life.

4. Emotions in the person with 'plate armour' are frozen. There is a palpable high-tension quality in the energy fields around the body. This allows the person to apparently build an effective, well-structured life. Physically they seem to be firm, well-built, with good muscular tone. The individual is however often unfulfilled due to a low level of sensitivity. Cardiac or ulcerative conditions may develop, as well as musculoskeletal problems such as tendonitis. While appearing to have a well ordered life, the lack of feeling often leads to a life-crisis, such as a coronary attack, which may prove a watershed for restructuring their life.

5. In some people an 'energy depletion' block exists in which the flow of energy to the ends of the limbs is drastically reduced (making it obvious during scanning) and resulting in weakness or even physical problems related to the limbs. The energy and physical alterations may be a metaphor for an inability to 'stand on their own two feet' in life or as a representation of a feeling of failure.

6. Finally there is the 'energy leak' where, instead of a smooth flow onwards from particular joints, energy seems to 'leak' from them. This may relate to an unconscious desire to be unable to respond to the environment or circumstances (based perhaps on a belief gained in childhood that response is dangerous or 'improper'). Physically it will relate to malcoordination or other physical (joint) abnormalities or problems. The limbs will be cold and may feel vulnerable. The leaking energy is palpable close to the joints in such limbs.

Brennan asks you to ask yourself which blocks you have used in your life as a result of early experience or conditioning?

Let us briefly return to the work of Fritz Smith M.D. (*Inner Bridges*) who gives this view of the energy body which Krieger, Joy and Brennan have shown us how to palpate in their respective ways:

> The working energy model of the human body is composed of three functional units: first, the non-organised background field of energy; second, the vertical movement of current conducted through the body which orients us to our environment; and third, the internal flows of the body which are produced because of the body's unique and individualised presence and which organise us into discrete functioning units. The last pattern – energy flow within the body – is further divided into three levels: the deep current through the bone and skeletal system; the middle currents through the soft tissues of the body; and the superficial level of vibration beneath the skin surface.

It is Smith's aim to make direct contact with these vibrational fields and he uses his unique 'bridging' methods (pressure, traction, bending, twisting or a non-moving fulcrum), as described in earlier chapters, to achieve this end. Via these means he assesses the clarity, density, pliability and other characteristics of energy, as well as the speed with which it responds (as evidenced by changes in rapid eye movement or breathing pattern for example) to such contact (or to needles in acupuncture).

Particular areas of energy dysfunction relate, he believes, to specific forms of mento-emotional discord. Thus sexual problems relate to the sacral area, security/insecurity to the pelvic bowl, power to the lumbar area, anger and frustration to the hips and jaw, compassion to the heart, sadness to the chest, creativity to the throat and intuition to the brow. He uses these generalizations (his word) to help assess the physical-emotional (or energetic) nature of the patient.

Richard Pavek has developed a system of 'physioemotional release therapy' called SHEN, which uses methods similar to those described in this chapter to release, or normalize, energy dysfunction (SHEN calls this biophysical) resulting from emotional stress. (*Handbook of SHEN: Physioemotional Release Therapy.*) He states that it is not difficult to feel the 'physioemotional' field, in the same ways described by Krieger, Joy and Brennan, in the palm of the scanning hand(s) as 'changes in temperature, tingles, prickles, pressure, "electricity" or "magnetism"'.

He amplifies these views as follows:

> The sensations [felt by the scanning hand] are usually different when the hand is over an area of physical pain, inflammation, tension and/or when release of emotion occurs when the hand is over an emotion region. The sensations picked up over an area of pain do not feel the same as the ones over a centre that is releasing emotion.

A series of exercises are given, some of which are the same as those already described in this (and previous) chapter(s), but with some useful variations.

Exercise 10. Do Exercise 1 again (feeling the 'bounce' of the energy field between the palms of your hands as you vary the distance between them) and after sensing the energy as a pressure, hold this and then begin to rotate your palms in small circles as though you were holding a ball between the palms, the hands travelling in a series of circular motions away and then towards yourself, one hand travelling forward as the other travels back, all the while keeping the palms facing each other, as far apart as you noted the sense of 'pressure'. The circles described should be about 10 inches in diameter.

Does the field change?

Pavek suggests that this process should alter the feel, as it 'energizes' the field, much as a nail stroked across a magnet will become energized. This is a useful way of enhancing sensitivity prior to performing energy balancing or diagnosis.

SHEN, as a system, demands a great deal of practice, as do all the practical applications of the methods touched on above. These few examples are by no means a complete representation of the depth of the work described by Krieger, Joy, Brennan, Smith or Pavel, being merely introductory concepts and exercises, which can be carried further if they trigger an interest.

Notes for the Enquiring Mind

Those who would like to explore this apparently uncharted area of healing further should also read the research work of L.E. Eeman as described in his book *Cooperative Healing*. Eeman was a pioneer studying human energy patterns who finally concluded:

> Do not the experiments described recall the aura so frequently described by occultists, mystics and clairvoyants? Do they not combine to suggest that there may, in fact, be, for right handers:
> a. a flow of electro-magnetic(?) force down the left and up the right side of the body (clockwise), and also
> b. clockwise inner vortices, and
> c. the reverse for left-handers? (p. 351).

He appeals for research to continue in this field since physical medicine has no evidence to offer on the subject.

Study should also be made of three other areas:

1. The Japanese system of Aikido, excellently explained in two books published by Japan Publications Inc *Ki in Daily Life* (Tokyo 1978) and *Book of Ki: Coordinating Mind and Body in Daily Life*. (Tokyo 1978).
2. The Chinese system of Qigong, explained in *The Wonders of Qigong*. Compiled by China Sports Magazine and published in Los Angeles by Wayfarer Publications in 1985.
3. Polarity Therapy, on which numerous books exist, including *Polarity Therapy* by Randolph Stone D.C. (published by the author, 1954) and *A Guide to Polarity Therapy* by Maruti Seidman, (Newcastle Publishing, North Hollywood, 1986).

Chapter 10

Palpation and Emotional States

Sherrington (*Man on His Nature*) asked in 1937, 'Can we stress too much that... any path we trace in the brain leads directly or indirectly to muscle?' Wilfred Barlow ('Anxiety and Muscle Tension Pain' *British Journal of Clinical Practice* Vol. 13, No. 5) stated in 1959, 'There is an intimate relationship between states of anxiety and observable (and therefore palpable) states of muscular tension.'

Use of electromyographic techniques has shown a statistical correlation between unconscious hostility and arm tension as well as leg muscle tension and sexual themes (R. Malmo, *Psychosomatic Medicine* 2, 9. 1949). Sainsbury (*J. Neurology, Neurosurgery and Psychiatry* 17, 3. 1954) showed that when 'neurotic' patients complained of feeling tension in the scalp muscles, there was electromyographic evidence of scalp muscle tension.

Wolff (in his famous book *Headache and Other Head Pains*) proved that the majority of patients with headache showed, 'marked contraction in the muscles of the neck...most commonly due to sustained contractions associated with emotional strain, dissatisfaction, apprehension and anxiety'.

Even thinking about activity produces muscular changes. In 1930 Jacobson (*Americal Journal of Physiology*, 91, 567) demonstrated 'It is impossible to conceive an activity without causing fine contractions in all those muscles which produce the activity in reality.'

Barlow sums up the emotion/muscle connection thus:

> Muscle is not only the vehicle of speech and expressive gesture, but has at least a finger in a number of other emotional pies – for example, breathing regulation, control of excretion, sexual functioning and above all an influence on the body schema through proprioception. Not only are emotional *attitudes*, say, of fear, and aggression mirrored immediately in the muscle, but also such moods as depression, excitement and evasion have their characteristic muscular patterns and postures.

Ford, in his book *Where Healing Waters Meet*, summarizes the early, less controversial, work of Wilhelm Reich, who rejected the exclusivity of the concepts that underlying physical conditions created the environment in which psychological dysfunction would occur, or that physical dysfunction was necessarily the result of psychological forces.

Rather he synthesized the two positions stating that: 'Muscular attitudes and character attitudes have the same function... They can replace one another and be influenced by one another. Basically they cannot be separated.'

As Ford puts it:

> When he encountered difficult psychological resistance (character armouring) in a patient, he moved to the corresponding areas of physical tension (muscular armouring) in the body, and used various forms of somatic therapy to correct the underlying physical distortions... Similarly if he was unable to affect a change in the tension of the patient's body through somatic therapy, he resorted to working with the psychological issues beneath the tension.

Palpation, insofar as it relates to emotional states, therefore requires the ability to observe (patterns of use, posture, attitudes, tics and habits) and feel for changes in the soft tissues which relate to emotionally charged states, acute or chronic. One of the key elements in this relates to breathing function which is intimately connected with emotion (see p. 204).

British osteopath Philip Latey has described patterns of distortion which coincide with particular clinical problems (*Muscular Manifesto*). He uses an analogy of 'three fists' because, he says, the unclenching of a fist correlates with physiological relaxation while the clenched fist indicates fixity, rigidity, overcontracted muscles, emotional turmoil, withdrawal from communication and so on:

> The lower fist is centred entirely on pelvic function. When I describe the upper fist I will include the head, neck, shoulders and arms with the upper chest throat and jaw. The middle fist will be focussed mainly on the lower chest and upper abdomen.

He describes the patient who enters the consulting room as showing an 'image posture', which is the impression the patient subconsciously wishes you to see, of him/her. If instructed to relax as far as possible the next image we see is that of 'slump posture', in which gravity acts on the body and it responds according to its unique attributes, tensions and weaknesses. Here it is common to observe overactive muscle groups coming into operation, hands, feet, jaw and facial muscles may writhe and clench or twitch.

Finally when the patient lies down and relaxes we come to the deeper image we wish to examine, the 'residual posture'. Here we find the tensions the patient cannot release. It is palpable and, says Latey, leaving aside sweat, skin and circulation, the deepest 'layer of the onion' available to examination.

What is seen varies from person to person according to their state of mind and well-being. Apparent is a record or psycho-physical pattern of the patient's responses, actions, transactions and interactions with his/her environment. The patterns of contraction which are found bear a direct relationship with the patient's unconscious, and provide a reliable avenue for discovery and treatment. They are providing sensory input to the patient and this is of considerable importance.

One of Latey's concepts involves a mechanism which leads to muscular contraction as a means of disguising a sensory barrage resulting from an emotional state. Thus he describes a sensation which might arise from the pit of the stomach being hidden by contraction of the muscles attached to the lower ribs, upper abdomen and the junction between the chest and lower spine; genital and anal sensations might be drowned out by contraction of hip, leg and low back musculature. Throat sensations might be concealed with contraction of the shoulder girdle, neck, arms and hands.

A restrained expression of emotion itself results in suppression of activity and ultimately chronic contraction of the muscles which would be used were these emotions expressed, be they rage, fear, anger, joy, frustration, sorrow or anything else. Latey points out that all areas of the body producing sensations which arouse emotional excitement may have their blood supply reduced by muscular contraction. Also sphincters and hollow organs can be held tight until numb. He gives as examples the muscles which surround the genitals and anus as well as the mouth, nose, throat, lungs, stomach and bowel.

In assessing these and other patterns of muscular tension in relation to emotional states Latey divides the body into three regions which he describes as the 'lower fist' (metaphor for a clenched fist) which centres entirely on pelvic function, the 'upper fist' which includes head, neck, shoulders, arms, upper chest, throat and jaw; and finally the middle fist which focuses mainly on the lower chest and upper abdomen.

Why are Latey's concepts so important? Because he comes close to an explanation of the mechanisms at work in the body-mind problems which are familiar to all who work on the human body with their hands. He avoids more conjectural explanations involving electro-magnetic energy, chakras, auras or energy fields or flows; not that such explanations are necessarily any less valid than Latey's, but he provides another way of seeing the problem.

Lower Fist

'The lower fist describes the muscular function of the pelvis, low back, lower abdomen, hips, legs and feet, with their mechanical, medical and psychosomatic significance.'

He identifies the central component of this region as the pelvic diaphragm, stretching as it does across the pelvic outlet, forming the floor of the abdominal cavity. The perineum allows egress for the bowel, vagina and urinary tract as well as the blood vessels and nerve supply for the genitalia. Each opening being controlled by powerful muscular sphincters which can be compressed by contraction of the muscular sheet.

When our emotions or feelings demand that we need to contract the pelvic outlet a further group of muscular units come into play which increases the pressure on the area from the outside. These are the muscles which adduct the thighs and which tilt the pelvis forwards and rotate the legs inwards, dramatically increasing compressive forces on the perineum, especially if the legs are crossed.

The impression this creates is one of 'closing in around the genitals' and is observed easily in babies and young children when anxious or in danger of wetting themselves. You can reproduce these contractions experimentally as follows:

Exercise 1. Stand upright, legs apart a little and exert maximum pressure and weight through the arches of the feet trying to flatten them to the floor. Sustain this effort for at least two minutes and sense the changes in your overall posture; feel the details of what is happening in the feet, knees, legs, hips, pelvis and spine. Feel the tensions begin to build around the pelvis and upper body parts. Note where discomfort begins.

If this sort of contraction is short lived no damage occurs. If it is prolonged and repetitive however, compensatory (adaptation stage) changes appear involving those muscles which abduct the legs, rotate them outwards and which pull the pelvis upright.

If the correction is incomplete the pelvis remains tilted forwards requiring additional contraction of low back muscles in order to maintain an erect posture.

Another pattern which is sometimes observed is of tension in the muscles of the buttocks which act to reinforce the perineal tension from behind. This tends to compress the anus more than the genitals and produces a different postural picture.

Exercise 2. Demonstrate this on yourself by standing and squeezing your anus tight, contracting the buttocks really hard and holding this for two or three minutes.

Feel the changes of posture and feelings of tension, strength and weakness in different parts of your body.

Problems of a mechanical nature which stem from the lower fist contraction include: internally rotated legs and 'knock-knees'; unstable knee joints; pigeon-toed stance resulting in flat arches. Here then is the onset of symptoms in 'knock-kneed, flat-footed children', and here also lies the answer.

The main mechanical damage is to the hip joints, due to compression and over-contraction of mutually opposed muscles. The hip is forced into its socket, muscles shorten and as there is loss of rotation and the ability to separate the legs, backward movement becomes limited. Uneven wear commences with obvious long-term end results. If this starts in childhood damage may include deformity of the ball and socket joint of the hip.

Low back muscles are also involved and this may represent the beginning of chronic backache, pelvic dysfunction, coccygeal problems and disc damage. The abdominal muscles are also affected since they are connected to changes in breathing function which result from the inability of the lower diaphragm to relax and allow proper motion to take place.

Medical complications which can result from these muscular changes involve mainly circulatory function since the circulation to the pelvis is vulnerable to stasis. Haemorrhoids, varicose veins, urethral constriction become more likely as do chances of urethritis and prostatic problems. All forms of gynaecological problems are more common and childbirth becomes more difficult as well.

Exercise 3. Assessing pelvic motion while patient is breathing.
1. Have the patient seated and feel for a gentle motion of the sacrum (pelvis) tipping forwards on inhalation and backwards on exhalation.
2. Patient side-lying, knees bent together, a hand over the sacrum allows pelvic breathing motion to be assessed. In good function there should be a slight lengthening of the lower body on inhalation and a shortening on exhalation.
3. Patient lies on back, knees and head supported a few inches from the surface. You sit at the side and rest your arm across the front of the pelvic bones, your hand resting on far hip, and feel for a rocking motion during respiration, as above.

In addition try resting the other hand just above the sacrum, under the patient at the same time. This helps the patient to become aware of the subtle respiratory motion of the sacrum/pelvis.

Exercise 4. Self treatment. If no such rhythmic motion is palpable (often the case) have the patient lie face down (or do this yourself), taking one arm back and down to cup their (your) own perineum. Practise feeling for the difference between normal relaxed motion of the phases of breathing when relaxed and the restricted pattern when they (you) clench the buttocks.

By breathing deeply in this position the abdomen is compressed against the floor or table and perineal motion is forced to occur. They (you) can learn to increase the excursion by relaxing the muscles of the region. This improves further if the tense muscles of the region are released by treatment. A profound weakness of the legs is often felt as relaxation of these muscles begins, and this may last for hours. As tension goes so vulnerability increases and reassurance is required. This is only a part of the restoration of normal function, but it is a beginning.

Middle Fist

When considering the middle fist Latey concentrates his attention on respiratory and diaphragm function and the many emotional inputs which affect this region. He discounts the popular misconception which states that breathing is produced by contraction of the diaphragm and the muscles which raise the rib cage, with exhalation being but a relaxation of these muscles. He states:

This is quite untrue. Breathing is produced by an active balance between the muscles mentioned above and the expiratory muscles that draw the rib-cage downwards and pull the ribs together. The even flow of easy breathing should be produced by dynamic interaction of these two sets of muscles.

The active exhalation phase of breathing is the result he suggests of:

1. Transversus thoracis which lies inside the front of the chest, attaching to the back of the sternum and fanning out inside the ribcage, and then continuing to the lower ribs where they separate. This is the inverted 'V' below the chest (it is known as transversus abdominis in this region). He calls this 'probably the most remarkable muscle in the body'. It has, he says, direct intrinsic abilities to generate all manner of uniquely powerful sensations, with even light contact sometimes producing reflex contractions of the whole body, or of the abdomen or chest and feelings of nausea and choking, all types of anxiety, fear, anger, laughter, sadness, weeping and so on.

The commonest sensations described by patients relating to its being touched include 'nausea, weakness, vulnerability and emptiness'. He discounts the idea that its sensitivity is related to the 'solar plexus', maintaining that its closeness to the internal thoracic artery is probably more significant, since when it is contracted it can exert direct pressure on it.

He believes that physiological breathing has as its central event a rhythmical relaxation and contraction of this muscle. Rigidity is often seen in the patient with 'middle fist' problems, where 'control' dampens the emotions which relate to it.

2. The other main exhalation muscle is serratus posterior inferior which runs from the upper lumbar spine, fanning upwards and outwards over the lower ribs which it grasps from behind, pulling them down and inwards on exhalation. These two muscles mirror each other, working together. Latey comments on the remarkable changes in tone in serratus relating to speech:

> The tone of this muscle varies with the emotional content of the patient's speech, especially when the emotions are highly labile and thinly veiled – near the surface. With the patients lying on their front the whole dorso-lumbar region may be seen to ripple in ridge-shaped patterns as they talk. As their words become progressively more 'loaded' the patterns become more emphatic. However it is more usual to find a static overcontracture of this muscle, with the underlying back muscles in a state of fibrous shortening and degeneration, reflecting the fixity of the transversus, and the extent of the emotional blockage.

Laughing, weeping and vomiting are three 'safety valve' functions of middle fist function which Latey is interested in. These are used by the body to help resolve internal imbalance. Anything stored internally which cannot be contained, emerges explosively via this route. In all three functions transversus alternates between full contraction and relaxation. In laughing and weeping there is a definite rhythm of contraction/relaxation of transversus, whereas in vomiting it remains in total contraction throughout each eliminative wave. Between waves of vomiting the breathing remains in the inspiratory phase, with upper chest panting. Transversus is slack in this phase.

Latey suggests that often it is only muscle fatigue which breaks cycles of laughter/weeping/vomiting, and he reminds us of phrases such as 'I wept or laughed until my sides ached'.

Nausea and vomiting are often associated with feelings such as 'I swallowed my pride' and 'stomaching an insult'.

He suggests seeking early feelings of hunger, need, fullness, emptiness, overfulness, nausea, rejection, expulsion and so on when working in this area, if we wish to uncover basic emotional links.

Latey delves into areas which are clearly within the realm of psychotherapy, and bodywork can be seen to have great importance in this field.

Exercise 5. In terms of assessing the function of the 'middle fist' he suggests that:

> With the patient balanced, sitting upright or lying sideways with knees up – the practitioner can easily learn the movements he is trying to encourage. The feelings of the middle fist disturbance surface most readily with the patient lying on their back. With one hand resting below the sternum (assessing transversus movement) the practitioner's other hand can feel the upper or lower fist movement. Nausea is often felt strongly in this position.

What might you notice in the patient as you hold this muscle? If they are feeling nauseous you might see a sudden pallor, sweat and protrusion of the chin followed by retching and gagging. A receptacle should be on hand and you should ask 'do you want to be sick?' After that you could ask 'what was stopping you?', for insights into underlying emotions.

If laughter is going to emerge this may be preceded by a squirming movement, a sideways look of 'naughtiness', superficial guilt, shame or embarrassment. A slight snort, snigger or grunt can lead to the main explosive laughter release. A comment such as 'It's ridiculous isn't it?' can help.

Before weeping starts the eyes become moist, the mouth quivers, a catch is heard in the voice. There is an expectation of encouragement and of comfort being offered. These emotions are inter-changeable and one may lead into another since these safety valves may be releasing feelings from quite different sources at the same time.

If panic starts it is characterized by a fluttering of the transversus, and is unmistakable. This can build into a shaking of the whole body, with breathing and chest movements becoming jerky and tremulous. Limbs twitch and eyes open wide. This sort of emotional explosion can have roots in very early experiences.

Latey pays great attention to the transversus muscle. He says, 'A feeling of tightness behind or below the breastbone marks the beginning of a cycle of emotion linked to this muscle (recrimination, pity, disgust etc). Is heartache an overtightness of the transversus muscle!'

As outlined above he encourages movement of the middle fist components (breathing and body work) and while doing so registers feelings of unease in the patient:

> Panic starts as a very definite fluttering of the transversus muscle itself and is quite unmistakable. Given full play it rapidly builds into a shaking of the whole body. The chest movements and breathing are jerky and tremulous: the limbs are twitchy: the eyes wide and staring in alarm. I have to look elsewhere for the meaning of panic: the chains of investigation are tortuous and difficult – invariably when fully exposed they lead back to earliest feelings.

The clinical problems associated with middle fist dysfunction relate to resulting distortions of blood vessels, internal organs, autonomic nervous system involvement and alteration in the neuro-endocrine balance. Diarrhoea, constipation, colitis may be involved but more direct results relate to lung and stomach problems. Thus bronchial asthma is an obvious example of middle fist fixation.

There is a typical associated posture with the shoulder girdle raised and expanded as if any letting go would precipitate a crisis. Compensatory changes usually include very taught deep neck and shoulder muscles. In treating such a problem Latey starts by encouraging function of the middle fist itself then extending into the neck and shoulder muscles, encouraging them to relax and drop, he then goes back to the middle fist. Dramatic expressions of alarm, unease and panic may be seen. The patient on discussing what they feel might report sensations of being smothered, drowned, choked, engulfed, crushed, obliterated. They relate to early life panic sensations and may go to the person's very core. 'Asthma is not easy to treat. Some merely require to mourn the loss (or lack) of motherly tenderness, soothing and comfort. Most have a great deal more work to do.'

When middle fist dysfunction involves digestive function this can involve postural alterations and emotional conflicts common in adolescents, says Latey.

> The lower end of the oesophagus passes through the muscular part of the diaphragm before joining the stomach. There is an intriguing mechanism which allows for the passage of food, or regurgitation of vomit, between the chest and the abdomen. When the diaphragm is contracted the muscular opening is constricted. In order to allow free flow it must be relaxed (full expiration) with the lower ribs pulled slightly together (transversus contraction).
>
> This device frequently fails when there is a chronic disturbance of the middle fist – the 'lower end of swallowing' is not happening properly. This may merely lead to wind, burping or fullness. However when the neuro-endocrine/smooth muscle activity is also disturbed the consequences may be more severe. Peptic ulcers, heartburn, reflux oesophagitis, hiatus hernia and so on are all medical conditions associated with middle fist problems. Here the filling and emptying of the stomach and duodenum, with their

internal secretions, have become chronically disordered.

We discussed briefly (p.225) Latey's methods for the holding and releasing of the middle fist and he suggests that this can lead to total or partial resolution of such dysfunction.

> However most patients only achieve partial resolution: when the middle fist disturbance begins to resolve the conflict is transferred to the mouth, neck and throat. Even though severe gastro-intestinal symptoms may have dissipated, we may still be left with a more complex problem involving the upper fist (the first part of swallowing).

If patients begin to weep, stopping and starting this process of release, Latey suggests the safety valve is only slightly open. He sees the pelvic and middle fist rhythms as coordinated but the head, neck and shoulders may seem rigid, fighting the movement. In such cases he has found that the situation can change dramatically by laying one's hands across the front of the patient's throat, a very light but firm touch which seems to effect sensitivity in the sterno-cleidomastoid muscles.

In such cases weeping may become full-bodied giving a total expression of grief with an orgasmic rhythm. Wailing and high-pitched crying may follow with expressions of complete misery and dejection, even leading to screams of terror. Unfettered rage, snapping and even biting is possible as the upper fist releases its pent-up tensions and expresses itself for the first time in years. Patently this is an area where many may not wish to venture. It is powerful and involves the need for nerves of steel on the part of the operator, however it is in such catharsis that healing may occur of pains and hurts buried for decades.

Upper Fist

The metaphor of the clenched fist, which is used to describe regions of the body associated with chronic, often emotionally based, contractions, is a powerful image. We have looked at the middle fist (diaphragm, respiratory muscles, abdomen) and also the lower fist which, not unnaturally, focused on the pelvic region (as well as low back and lower abdomen, hips, legs and feet).

The upper fist involves muscles which extend from the thorax to the back of the head, where the skull and spine join, extending sideways to include the muscles of the shoulder girdle. These muscles therefore set the relative positions of the head, neck, jaw, shoulders and upper chest, and to a large extent the rest of the body follows this lead (it was F.M. Alexander who showed that the head-neck relationship is the primary postural control mechanism). This region, says Latey, almost with relish, is 'the centre, *par excellence*, of anxieties, tensions and other amorphous expressions of unease'.

In chronic states of disturbed upper fist function, he asserts, the main physical impression is one of restrained, over-controlled, damped down expression. The feeling of the muscles is that they are controlling an 'explosion of affect'. In contrast to the lower fist which impresses us with its grip on sensual functions, the upper fist has contracted in response to, or to restrain response to, the outer world.

Just what it is that is being restrained is never obvious from the muscles themselves, but interpreting facial muscles may give a clue. Far more important though than the expressions on the face are those which have been withheld. Those experiences which are not allowed free play on the face are expressed in the muscles of the skull and the base of the skull. This is he believes of central importance in problems of headache, especially migraine. Says Latey, 'I have never seen a migraine sufferer who has not lost complete ranges of facial expression, at least temporarily.'

The mechanical consequences of upper fist fixations are many and varied, ranging from stiff neck to compression factors leading to disc degeneration and facet wear. Swallowing and speech difficulties are common as are shoulder dysfunctions including brachial neuritis, Reynaud's syndrome and carpel tunnel problems.

He states,

> The medical significance of upper fist contracture is mainly circulatory. Just as lower fist contraction contributes to circulatory stasis in the legs, pelvis, perineum and lower abdomen; so may upper fist contracture have an even more profound effect. The blood supply to the head, face, special sense, the mucosa of the nose, mouth, upper respiratory tract, the heart itself and the main blood vessels are controlled by the sympathetic nervous system and its main 'junction boxes' (ganglia) lie just to the front of the vertebrae at the base of the neck.

Thus headaches, eye pain, ear problems, nose and throat as well as many cardiovascular troubles may contain strong mechanical elements relating to upper fist muscle contractions.

He reminds us that it is not uncommon for cardiovascular problems to manifest at the same time as chronic muscular shoulder pain (avascular necrosis of the rotator cuff tendons) and that the longus colli muscles are often centrally involved in such states.

He looks to the nose, mouth, lips, tongue, teeth, jaws and throat for evidence of functional change related to upper fist dysfunction, with relatively simple psychosomatic disturbances underlying these. Sniffing, sucking, biting, chewing, tearing, swallowing, gulping, spitting, dribbling, burping, vomiting, sound-making and so on are all significant functions which might be disturbed acutely or chronically. *And as with middle and lower fist dysfunction these can all be approached via breathing function.*

> When all the components of the upper fist are relaxed, the act of expiration produces a noticeable rhythmical movement. The neck lengthens, the jaw rises slightly (rocking the whole head), the face fills out, the upper chest drops.
>
> When the patient is in difficulty I may try to encourage these movements by manual work on the muscles and gentle direction to assist relaxed expiration. Again, by asking the patient to let go and let feelings happen, I encourage resolution. Specific elements often emerge quite readily,

especially those mentioned with the middle fist, the need to vomit, cry, scream, etc.

In relation to headache Latey observes:

> We can often see the headache to be a more general avoidance mechanism. The way in which the generalised focus of pain occupies attention is significant. It clouds and limits concept formation and observation. There is always a deadening and coarsening of sensation and expressiveness. It seems as though the patient uses the headache to hold some perturbation at bay until it can be coped with more responsively, or disappears.
>
> With more severe migraines, with disturbances of vision and nausea, it is often necessary to work through feelings of disgust in considerable detail. Fear of poisoning may be a strong component of nausea, and usually dates back to earliest disturbances of feeling.

He also spends time analysing shock and withdrawal experienced in early months of life as life's realities are recoiled from. This leads, he believes, to our failing to learn from experience as we flinch from emotionally unpleasant episodes.

Withdrawal characteristics determine many of his clinical perspectives. Superficially at any rate they are easy to recognize:

> The dull lifeless tone of the flesh; lifeless flaccidity of larger surface muscle (or spastic rigidity); lifeless hard fibrous state of deep residual postural muscles (with the possible exception of the head and neck muscles); the over-investment of the person in his eyes and ears - hearing and seeing.

More profound pointers to withdrawal are more subtle:

> The ritualised expression of any 'emotion' in a depersonalised and unspontaneous fashion; the use of language that denies the central presence of unity of self, wards off threats (from outside or inside temptation perhaps) and grasps hold of common insanities of our civilisation. These insanities are greatly worsened by social/family mystification (studied by R.D. Laing *et al*).

Exercise 6. Examine someone with known emotional stress symptoms and see whether you can identify patterns of muscular change as outlined above; dull lifeless, lifeless flaccidity, spastic rigidity, lifeless hard fibrous and so on; or breathing dysfunction as described earlier in this chapter.

Look also for 'ritualised expression of emotion' or 'use of language that denies central presence and unity of self, wards off threats', lack of facial expression - which ones are missing? - and also statements about bodily feelings that seem unusual.

Latey suggests that we consider three 'fists', or regions, of abnormal tension, contraction and restriction as we try to look and feel for the physical manifestations of emotional turmoil. A variation on precisely this same theme is found in the methods grouped together as Somatosynthesis. This is described quite beautifully in Clyde Ford's book *Where Healing Waters Meet*.

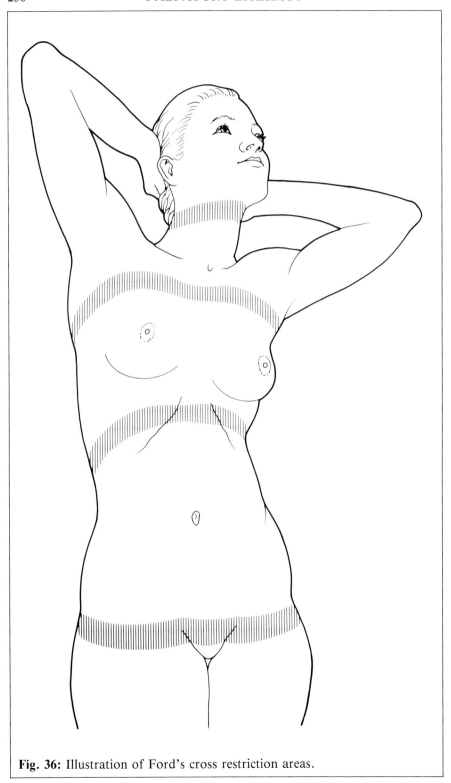

Fig. 36: Illustration of Ford's cross restriction areas.

He believes that, 'There is a close relationship between the diagnostic and therapeutic uses of touch. When touch is involved (palpation), it is not uncommon to hear of the diagnosis turning into therapy without the awareness of the therapist or the patient.' He continues: 'My approach to therapeutic touch has always been to keep it simple, getting maximal results from minimal number of techniques and procedures.'

Which areas does he work on in dealing with emotional problems? 'I might begin by working with the four major areas of cross-restriction in the body; the base of the pelvis [Latey's lower fist], the base of the rib cage [Latey's middle fist], the base of the neck and the base of the skull [together these are Latey's upper fist].'

It is in these regions, he asserts, that the usual orientation of soft tissues in a vertical direction are different, they are horizontally directed:

> Usually the horizontal tissue cross-restricts the vertical tissue of the body, thereby hampering normal muscle movement, fluid flow and nerve transmission. *The practical result is that these areas turn out to be the places that most of us experience and retain stress, tension and pain in our bodies. And they are also the areas often related to the deeper psychological issues beneath our physical signs and symptoms. A simple straightforward approach to working with these cross-restrictions is to gently compress them from front to back.* [My emphasis.]

How does he palpate and treat these (and other) dysfunctions? 'Seasoned palpators have long known that the best hand is a light hand – the lighter the touch, the more information can be obtained.' It is by lightly palpating, projecting the sense of touch, and being receptive to whatever information radiates into the hand that he identifies areas of maximal tension and dysfunction:

> Once I have palpated to determine where to touch (therapeutically), there are three things I take into account: depth, direction and duration. How deep does my touch need to be? Should it be at the level of the energy field where no physical contact is involved, at the skin surface...or pressing firmly into the (patient's) body.

He then decides in which direction this contact should move, straight down, right, left, pulling, pushing, steady or continuous movement or a combination of these? And finally he allows the tissues themselves to determine how long the force should be held.

Wolf's final thought, that we 'remember that palpation and therapy are happening simultaneously', should be one of our key considerations throughout our work. We can now see that Latey and Wolf approach these problems with slightly different methods, as does Marion Rosen whose work is considered next.

The Rosen Method

Marion Rosen, a brilliant physical therapist, has evolved a method which addresses the same physical manifestations of emotional turmoil as Latey's approach. (*Rosen Method* by Elaine Mayland Ph.D.). 'Rosen Method is not a mechanical process. It is a journey taken together by client and practitioner towards self-discovery.'

The practitioner observes the patient's back:

- Are the muscles tense?
- Where does breath move freely?
- Where is it withheld?
- What statement is the patient making with his body?
- What has to happen so that he can relinquish that contracted space?
- What is the direction in which the muscles are holding?
- Does this holding bear down, hold him together, puff him up or separate the top from the bottom of the body by tightening in the middle? (Latey's middle fist).

Exercise 7. Examine someone (if possible the person used in Exercise 6) with known emotional stress symptoms and see whether you can identify any such patterns. Compare these with the findings from Exercise 6. The hands are then run gently over the back muscles seeking information, comparing what was observed with what is palpated.

The task is to increase patient awareness of areas of 'holding' in a non-judgemental manner. As areas are palpated and held so alterations slowly manifest as the patient becomes aware, breathes into those restricted regions as the practitioner 'Watches and feels for the place on the back that is most unmoving, held, or not included in his expression of himself. He is unaware that he is holding back.'

Exercise 8. Palpate and observe the back muscles of a prone patient with known emotional problems. Take time to locate the most restricted muscular area of the back and hold a palpating hand against it, meeting its tension, just taking out the slack. Observe what happens a) to these tissues over a period of some minutes, and b) what changes, if any, take place in the breathing pattern.

The practitioner's task is to follow such tissues as they release and relax, continuing until all the back is released and breathing function is freely observed in all the tissues. Then attention turns to the diaphragm and anterior surface. This major breathing muscle reveals tensions being held and changes in its function are readily palpated, at the same time as facial expression alterations are seen.

Compare a description of what might be observed when the Rosen method is used with the description given by Latey on p.226.

Sometimes as the practitioner works with the muscles that move the diaphragm, a flutter of the diaphragm itself can be seen. Movements in the abdomen might begin as they do when a person is sobbing or crying, although the expression on the face has not changed, leading her [the practitioner] to believe that the sadness that is being expressed in the body is not reaching the face and the consciousness of the client.

Other tensions, in the neck or chest perhaps, are then sought which are specifically palpated and worked on until emotional release occurs. The work is accompanied by careful observation and skilled questioning. As should be clear the process of palpation is in fact the start of the treatment process (something which can also be said for Lief's Neuromuscular Technique).

The essence of this approach is the identification via observation and palpation of restricted areas in which the breathing function fails to manifest itself. Until this is achieved subsequent release is not easily achieved. As Mayland says:

> All we want is for a person to get connected with what they are holding back. The degree to which they repress, that they will not allow themselves to experience, that they carry around with them...form a barrier to our living. They are like loads, like rocks in our being.

It is perhaps helpful to note that the amount of pressure used on tense 'held' areas, when Rosen Method is applied, is very similar to that described by Fritz Smith and Stanley Lief in earlier chapters. It 'meets' the muscle, not attempting to overwhelm it or make it do anything. Awareness is the key, with release occurring from the patient's side not as a forced event.

In Rosen Method, as in Latey's work, there is a hierarchy of emotions, linked to specific areas:

- Deep fear and deep love are associated with the region of the pelvis (or deep in the belly) and where the legs meet the pelvis.
- Repressed anger and sadness are often found in the upper torso or neck.
- Feelings towards others relate to the middle trunk and heart area.
- Fear and anxiety are repressed around the diaphragm.
- Anger, sadness and fear are, according to Marion Rosen, easier to release than love.

Rosen Method is characterized by the gentleness of the approach. Emotions are re-experienced, not forced, as the client learns that feelings are just feelings and not the events which precipitated their being locked away. The method leads to self-acceptance and release from long-held tensions, identified by palpation and observation.

Upledger's somatoemotional release (*Craniosacral Therapy*) described in earlier chapters, is worthy of further mention at this point; using gentle compressive or traction forces (slight inferiorly directed compressive force upon parietals of the seated patient, compressing cervical and thoracic vertebrae caudally; gentle medial compression of anterior ilia with patient standing; grasping ankles of supine patient and introducing slight compressive or traction force and so on). Upledger requires the therapist to follow the 'unwinding' process which the body then initiates.

Palpatory and proprioceptive skills of a high order are required to achieve this, since not only are the hands required to follow the slow unwinding process but also to register and prevent any tendency for the unwinding to follow a repetitive pathway.

While this method is used largely to release locked-in trauma-induced forces, 'repressed emotional components of the somatic injury are frequently and concurrently released'. Panic or hysteria related to the trauma are relived and adaptational energy released.

Upledger warns: 'Be alert. Do not inhibit your patient by dragging on their body movements. Try to follow where the patient's body leads you.' The patient may finally adopt the position in which the trauma occurred.

While somatoemotional release (as in Rosen Method) seems to describe therapy rather than palpation/diagnosis, the distinction is essentially blurred when these approaches are used as described by their developers. Palpation skills determine the practitioners ability to perform these therapeutic methods.

Bibliography

Adams, Steinnetz, Heisey, Holmes and Greenman, 'Physiologic basis for skin properties in palpatory physical diagnosis', *Journal of the American Osteopathic Association*, Feb 1982.

Paul Van Allen, *1963 Yearbook Academy of Applied Osteopathy*.

Paul Van Allen, *1964 Yearbook Academy of Applied Osteopathy*.

Beryl Arbuckle, *Selected Writings of Beryl Arbuckle*, National Osteopathic Institute and Cerebral Palsy Foundation, 1977.

H. Bailey and C. Beckwith, *1966 Yearbook Academy of Applied Osteopathy*.

W. Barlow, 'Anxiety and Muscle Tension Pain', *British Journal of Clinical Practice*, 13, 5.

J.P. Barral and P. Mercier, *Visceral Manipulation*, Eastland Press, 1988.

Myron Beal, 'Palpatory testing of somatic dysfunction in patients with cardiovascular disease', *Journal of the American Osteopathic Association*, July 1983.

Alan Becker, 'Parameters of resistance', *1973 Yearbook Academy of Applied Osteopathy*.

Rollin Becker, *1963 Yearbook Academy of Applied Osteopathy*.

Rollin Becker, *1964 Yearbook Academy of Applied Osteopathy*.

Rollin Becker, *1965 Yearbook Academy of Applied Osteopathy*.

I. Bischof and G. Elmiger, 'Connective tissue massage' in S. Licht (ed.) *Massage Manipulation and Traction*, Licht, New Haven 1960.

Blower and Griffin, *Ann Rhem Dis.* 1984.

Jean Bossy, 'Morphological data concerning acupuncture points and channel networks', *Acupuncture and Electrotherapeutics Research International Journal*, 9, 1984.

Barbara Ann Brennan, *Hands of Light*, Bantam 1987.

A. Brugger, 'Pseudo radikulare syndrome', *Acta Rheumatol*, 18, 1, 1960.

Butler and Gifford, *Physiotherapy*, Nov 1989.

R. Cailliet, *Low Back Pain Syndrome*, Blackwell, 1962.

Leon Chaitow, *Soft Tissue Manipulation*, Thorsons, 1988.

Leon Chaitow, *Instant Pain Control*, Thorsons, 1983.

Gerald Cooper, 'Clinical considerations of fascia in diagnosis and treatment', *1977 Yearbook of Applied Osteopathy*.

Bertrand De Jarnette, *Reflex Pain*, Nebraska 1934.

P. Diakow, 'Thermographic imaging of myofascial trigger points', *Journal of Manipulative and Physiologic Therapeutics*, 11, 2, 1988.

Jiri Dvorak, Vaclav Dvorak, *Manual Medicine: Diagnostics*, Georg Thiem Verlag, N.Y. 1984.

R. Ehrlinghauser 'Circulation of CSF through the connective tissue system', *1959 Yearbook Academy of Applied Osteopathy*.

H. Fryett, *Principles of Osteopathic Technic*, National Printing Co, Kirksville, 1954.

Viola Frymann, *1963 Yearbook of the Academy of Applied Osteopathy*.

Viola Frymann, 'Palpation', *1963 Yearbook of Selected Osteopathic Papers*.

R. Gerber, *Vibrational Medicine*, Bear and Co. 1988.

F. Goodheart, *Applied Kinesiology Workshop Manual*, 21 Edn, 1985.

J. Goldthwaite, *Essentials of Body Mechanics*, J.B. Lippencott, Philadelphia 1945.

Philip Greenman, *Principles of Manual Medicine*, Williams and Wilkins, 1989.

Gregory Grieve, *Mobilisation of the Spine*, Churchill Livingstone, 1984.

Laurie Hartmann, *Handbook of Osteopathic Technique*, Hutchinson, 1985.

Marshall Hoag, *Osteopathic Medicine*, McGraw Hill, 1969.

H.V. Hoover, 'A method for teaching functional technique', *1969 Yearbook of Academy of Applied Osteopathy*.

E. Jacobson, *Americal Journal of Physiology*, 91, 1930.

Vladimir Janda, 'Muscles, central nervous motor regulation and back problems' in I. Korr (ed.), *Neurobiological Mechanisms in Manipulative Therapy*, Plenum, 1977.

Vladimir Janda, *Muscle Function Testing*, Butterworths, 1983.

Vladimir Janda, 'Pain in the locomotor system', in Glasgow E. *et al.* (eds), *Aspects of Manipulative Therapy*, Churchill Livingstone, 1985.

William Johnston, 'Segmental Definition I, II', *Journal of the American Osteopathic Association*, Jan & Feb 1988.

Lawrence Jones, 'Strain/counterstrain', *Academy of Applied Osteopathy*, Colorado Springs 1981.

Brugh Joy, *Joy's Way*, J.P. Turner inc. 1979.

Deane Juhan, *Job's Body*, Station Hill Press, N.Y. 1987.

R. Kappler, 'Role of psoas mechanism in low-back complaints', *Journal of the American Osteopathic Association*, 72, April 1973.

E. Keller, M. Bzdek, 'Effects of Therapeutic Touch on tension headache pain', *Cooperative Connections*, X.2 Spring 1989.

J. Kellgren, *Clinical Science*, 3, 175, 1938; 4, 35, 1939.

Irvin Korr, *The Physiological Basis of Osteopathic Medicine*, Postgraduate Institute of Osteopathic Medicine and Surgery, N.Y. 1970.

Irvin Korr, 'Spinal cord as organizer of the disease process', *1976 Yearbook of Academy of Applied Osteopathy*.

Irvin Korr, *Journal of American Osteopathic Association*, Feb 1986.

Irvin Korr, 'Spinal cord as organizer of the disease process' Part 4, 'Axonal transport and neurotrophic function in relation to somatic dysfunction', *Academy of Applied Osteopathy*, March 1981.

D. Krieger, *The Therapeutic Touch*, Prentice Hall 1979.

Philip Latey, *Muscular Manifesto*, Latey, London 1980.

Karel Lewit, 'Muscular patterns in thoraco-lumbar lesions', *Manual Medicine*, 1986, 2.

Karel Lewit, *Manipulation in Rehabilitation of the Motor System*, Butterworths, 1987.

Harold Magoun, 'Osteopathic diagnosis and therapy for the general practitioner', *Journal of the American Osteopathic Association, Dec. 1948*.

G. Maitland, *Vertebral Manipulation*, Butterworths 1986.

R. Malmo, *Psychosomatic Medicine*, 2, 9, 1949.

E. Mayland, *Rosen Method*, Mayland, Palo Alto 1980.

R. McFarlane Tilley, 'Spinal stress patterns', *1961 Yearbook Academy of Applied Osteopathy*.

Carl McConnell, *The Practice of Osteopathy*, McConnell, 1899.

R. Melzack and P. Wall, *The Challenge of Pain*, Penguin, 1988.

J. Mennell, *Back Pain*, T. & A. Churchill, 1964.

F. Mitchell, *1976 Yearbook of the American Academy of Osteopathy*.

F. Mitchell, *Journal of the American Osteopathic Association June 1976*.

F. Mitchell, P. Moran and N. Pruzzo, *An Evaluation of Osteopathic Muscle Energy Procedure*, Valley Park, 1979.

Marsh Morrison, *Lecture Notes*, London 1969.

Roger Newman Turner, *Naturopathic Medicine*, Thorsons, 1984.

Raymond Nimmu, *Lecture Notes*, 1966.

Nordenstrom, *Biologically Closed Electric Circuits: Clinical, Experimental and Theoretical Evidence for an Additional Circulatory System*, Nordic Medical Publications, Stockholm 1983.

Charles Owens, *An Endocrine Interpretation of Chapman's Reflexes*, Academy of Applied Osteopathy, 1963.

R. Pavek, *Handbook of SHEN: Physioemotional Release Therapy*, SHEN Institute, California 1987.

Ida Rolf, *Rolfing: The Integration of Human Structures*, Harper and Row, 1977.

Hugo Rosers *et al.* 'Correlation of palpatory observations with the anatomic locus of acute myocardial infarction', *Journal of the American Osteopathic Association*, Feb 1971.

P. Sainsbury, *Journal of Neurology, Neurosurgery and Psychiatry*, 17, 3, 1954.

Hans Selye, *The Stress of Life*, McGraw-Hill, 1984.

Fritz Smith, *Inner Bridges: A Guide to Energy Movement and Body Structure*, Humanics New Age 1986.

A. Speransky, *A Basis for the Theory of Medicine*, International Publishers, N.Y. 1944.

W. Strachan, *1966 Yearbook Academy of Applied Osteopathy*.

W.G. Sutherland, *The Cranial Bowl*, The Osteopathic Cranial Association.

Sara Sutton, 'An osteopathic method of history taking and physical examination', *1977 Yearbook of Academy of Applied Osteopathy*.

J. Travell, D. Simons, *The Trigger Point Journal*, Williams & Wilkins, 1986.

J. Upledger and Vredevoogd, *Craniosacral Therapy*, Eastland Press, 1983.

J. Upledger, *Craniosacral Therapy II: Beyond the Dura*, Eastland Press, 1987.

D. Varma, *The Human Machine and its Forces*, Health for All Publications, London, 1905.

William Walton, 'Palpatory diagnosis of the osteopathic lesion', *Journal of the American Osteopathic Association*, Aug 1971.

George Webster, *1947 Yearbook of the American Academy of Osteopathy*.

P. Williams, *Lumbosacral spine*, McGraw Hill, 1965.

H. Wolff, *Headache and Other Head Pain*, Oxford University Press, 1948.

Yuan Curxin *et al.* 'Curative effect and mechanism of acupoints Pishu and Weishu', *Journal of Traditional Chinese Medicine*, 6, 4, 1986.

INDEX